M A P :
The Co-Creative
White Brotherhood
Medical Assistance Program

MAP

THE CO-CREATIVE
WHITE BROTHERHOOD
MEDICAL
ASSISTANCE
PROGRAM

MACHAELLE SMALL WRIGHT

PERELANDRA, LTD.

CENTER FOR NATURE RESEARCH
JEFFERSONTON ☞ VIRGINIA

"MAP" and "Co-Creative White Brotherhood Medical Assistance
Program" are trademarks of Perelandra, Ltd.

This book is manufactured in the United States of America.
Designed by Machaelle Small Wright and James F. Brisson.
Cover design by James F. Brisson, Williamsville, VT 05362
Editing by David and Machaelle Small Wright.
Mechanical editing by Albert Schatz, Ph.D.
Copyediting by Beverly Beane, Antrim, NH 03440.
Legwork, computer tech lifesaver, & meals by Clarence N. Wright.
Formatting, typsetting and computer wizardry
by Machaelle Small Wright.

This book was formatted, laid out and produced on an
AST Premium 286 computer using
the Xerox Ventura Publisher software along with
the Canon LBP-4 printer with an Eicon Laser Printer Adapter.

Printed on recycled paper.

Published by Perelandra, Ltd.,
P.O. Box 3603, Warrenton, VA 22186

Library of Congress Card Catalog Number: 90-063950
Wright, Machaelle Small
MAP: The Co-Creative White Brotherhood
Medical Assistance Program

ISBN 0-927978-05-9

4 6 8 9 7 5

Table of Contents

Preface

The Light at the End of the Tunnel

by Albert Schatz, Ph.D.*

This is an extraordinary book. To do it justice, I must begin by putting it in proper perspective. Man's localized destruction of nature has been responsible for the extinction of many animal species. Now our global assault on nature threatens *our* survival. Instead of implementing Franklin Delano Roosevelt's Four Freedoms, we have chosen a collision course with the Four Horsemen of the Apocalypse. Individuals who exhibit such self-destructive behavior are considered to be mentally deranged. But, like Thespians in a Greek tragedy, "merrily we go to hell."

We are running out of natural resources, out of natural environment, out of space, and out of time. In our suicidal assault on nature, we are approaching the point of no return. The world's military budget is a

* Dr. Schatz discovered the antibiotic Streptomycin, which was the first effective means of treating human tuberculosis. For this and other research, he received honorary degrees and medals, and was named an honorary member of scientific, medical and dental societies in Europe, Latin America and the U.S.

barometer, odometer, and speedometer of our mad rush to oblivion. The arms race turns out to have been a race to annihilation. The insanity of Vietnam has metastasized into global insanity. In Vietnam, "we had to destroy a city in order to save it." Now we are destroying the world allegedly to save it in one way or another, for one purpose or another. The wages of this sin were pointed out by Dwight Eisenhower in his 1953 Cross of Iron speech.

> . . . *Every gun that is made, every warship launched, every rocket fired signifies, in the final sense, a theft from those who hunger and are not fed, those who are cold and are not clothed.*
>
> *This world in arms is not spending money alone.*
>
> *It is spending the sweat of its laborers, the genius of its scientists, the hopes of its children.*
>
> *The cost of one modern heavy bomber is this: a modern brick school in more than thirty cities . . .*
>
> *We pay for a single fighter plane with a half million bushels of wheat.*
>
> *We pay for a single destroyer with new homes that could have housed more than eight thousand people.*
>
> *This, I repeat, is the best way of life to be found on the road the world has been taking.*
>
> *This is not a way of life at all, in any true sense. Under the cloud of threatening war, it is humanity hanging from a cross of iron . . .*

We obviously will not be saved by our anthropocentric science which has given us chemical dumps, deadly radioactive waste that we do not know how to dispose of, air and water pollution, carcinogenic pesticides and food additives, ineffective and harmful synthetic drugs, nerve gas, nuclear weapons, biological warfare, the profligate waste of nature resources, the global devastation of nature, and much more. This is what science means to many people. We obviously also will not be saved by academic scientists whose research is supported by grants from and, in turn, supports the pharmaceutical, agricultural, and chemical industries—and the military. Indeed, the military-industrial complex which Eisenhower warned us about has metastasized into a military-industrial-educational complex.

YE SHALL KNOW THE TRUTH
AND THE TRUTH SHALL MAKE YOU FREE

Where can we go from here? Is there a way out? I am convinced that our only salvation is what Machaelle Small Wright calls "co-creative science." This involves our consciously establishing a co-creative partnership with nature. But, before we do that, we should know what nature is and who we are with respect to nature.

This and other essential information is now readily available as a result of research that Machaelle has done in collaboration with nature. Her published reports are not merely descriptive narratives of devas, nature spirits, and other intelligences. Instead, they provide us with clear definitions and a simple hands-on approach so we know how and with whom we can communicate and work. Moreover, we can all engage in co-creative science and work in a co-creative partnership with nature, *if* we want to. It is not necessary that we take courses in biology, chemistry, physics, geology, calculus, etc. and get degrees. The only credentials we need are intent, sincerity, commitment, and the information and processes available in Perelandra publications.

Co-creative science is qualitatively different from the science we know because it integrates the involutionary input of nature (order, organization and life vitality/action) with the evolutionary dynamic of man (direction and purpose). Until now, science has been essentially evolutionary. (These and other terms are defined in Machaelle's publications.) Co-creative science is therefore not a linear advance over present-day science, but it is qualitatively unique. It was developed *de novo* in the sense that it is not derived from contemporary science. It employs different methodologies and obtains information from sources with which contemporary science has never worked. Co-creative science may be graphically represented, using the "V" diagram shown on the next page.

I believe that co-creative science is the science of the future, that it will revolutionize our understanding of science, philosophy, and psychology; and that it will provide us with a new kind of agriculture and new ways of achieving health.

This leads directly to Machaelle's book, *MAP: The Co-Creative White Brotherhood Medical Assistance Program.* All of us are concerned with health. But what is health? And

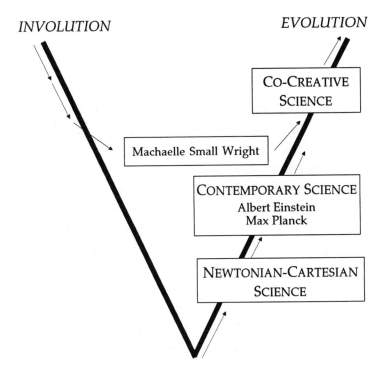

Newtonian-Cartesian Science, also known as Classical Science, developed in the 17th century. That science was based on the work of the physicist Sir Isaac Newton and the philosopher René Descartes. Contemporary, present-day science is based on the research of Max Planck, "the father of quantum mechanics" (1900), and Albert Einstein's theories of relativity (1905 and 1916).

how is it best achieved, supported, and maintained? Unfortunately, there is something wrong with how these questions are answered. While we have been bombarded with more and more information on health, our health has been declining. While we have been spending more and more money on health, we have become more and more unhealthy. Obviously, what we need is a new approach, one that will be effective. *MAP*, like

Machaelle's book *Flower Essences,* provides precisely that.

MAP is not allopathy, homeopathy, naturopathy, or any other conventional medical specialty. Nor is it related to alternative health modalities or holistic health. And it is not esoteric, occult, new age, or spiritual. All those approaches to health are essentially evolutionary developments by man.

MAP is qualitatively different because, like co-creative science of which it is a part, it integrates the involutionary input of nature with man's evolutionary development. The healthy human being is a balanced combination of these two dynamics. We do not need to know anatomy, physiology, biochemistry, pathology, psychology, etc. to use MAP effectively. As in the case of co-creative science, the only credentials we need are intent, sincerity, commitment, and the information and processes in Machaelle's book.

But *MAP* offers much more than health *per se.* Like Machaelle's other books, *MAP* also increases our understanding of who and what we are, what nature and reality are, what our place in the universe is, what our responsibilities are, and what amazing opportunities we have.

Machaelle's co-creative research with nature is not only the light at the end of the tunnel. It is also the entrance to the tunnel and the tunnel itself.

M A P :
The Co-Creative
White Brotherhood
Medical Assistance Program

L'Chaim

Chapter 1

Some Personal Comments and How MAP Was Developed

In 1982, my work expanded in ways that were both exhilarating and extremely challenging. Since 1976, I had been working exclusively with nature intelligences in research dedicated to developing a working partnership between humans and nature. But in 1982, I learned from nature that I could expand the research in a way that would link it directly into the activities of an organization called the "White Brotherhood." I also learned that this connection was beneficial to nature and to us, as well as to the White Brotherhood. So, I decided to do it.

This decision set off a chain of events that, among other things, led me into a whole new level of understanding of the human body and its relationship to the soul. You see, my decision to expand the research at Perelandra was a soul decision. Once the decision was made, I discovered that implementing it depended on my ability to physically hold, support and process all that the expansion required of me. I had understood

1

something about this relationship between the soul and the body for years, but the 1982 expansion brought it into a new and more intense light.

Usually, when I have discussed this situation with others, they immediately think that the thing one must do in order to meet the challenges of expansion is change the diet. Over the years, I've realized how much we lean on diet as a solution for everything. Well, I never changed my diet nor, after much questioning, was I ever instructed to change my diet. The eating patterns that I had established prior to 1982 were sufficient for what I was faced with after 1982. If diet wasn't the answer to my functioning well on this more expanded level of the nature research, then I would have to find other answers.

To help you to understand the scope of the expansion I am talking about and why it presented challenges, let me give you a thumbnail description of the White Brotherhood. After all, if you decide to enter the MAP program, you will be working with them as well, and I'm sure you'd appreciate knowing who they are. Before you get nervous, however, and think that your working with them will necessitate your dealing with the kinds of challenges I encountered, let me assure you that this will not be the case. I had to expand myself *into their dimension* in order to work with them on a daily basis in a working team relationship. This has impacted the scope, quality, direction and expression of the Perelandra work. Your expansion will center around your decision to work with the White Brotherhood in areas involving your health and personal balance. You will not have to expand into another dimension. In short, the White Brotherhood will be making "house calls."

I became aware of the White Brotherhood's link with the research at Perelandra in 1980. For two years, I ignored them while I maintained my focus on nature intelligences and our work exclusively. I figured that whatever connection the White Brotherhood had would be best handled by them and they didn't need me. Besides, at that time, I knew next to nothing about them and had no desire to know more.

Much has been written about the White Brotherhood, but I've thought a lot of it was garbage. Some people have felt or said that they are the sole "channellers" of the White Brotherhood, and this simply isn't true. The Brotherhood is a huge organization that is constantly connected to us in general and to many of us individually. It's just that usually they are only able to work with us on an intuitive level, and our link with them is unconscious on our part.

The Brotherhood is a large group of highly evolved souls dedicated to assisting the evolutionary process of moving universal reality, principles, laws and patterns through all planes and levels of form. They hold the major patterning and rhythms now being utilized for the shift we are all going through from the Piscean to the Aquarian era. When we link with them, they support and assist us by assuring that any work we do maintains its forward evolutionary motion and its connection to the new Aquarian dynamics.

They exist beyond time and history. I first heard about them during my stay at Findhorn in 1977. St. Germain, who had a close relationship with several Findhorn members, was referred to often and described as being a master teacher from the White Brotherhood. I was also told that the Order of the Melchizedek was a part of the Brotherhood, and it is from this group that all of the major religious leaders come who have been a part of our history. As I have said, I ignored the Brotherhood and its existence for years, assuming that they knew how to do their job, whatever that was, very well without me and that my focus was primarily on nature, not on human-oriented evolution. After all, this is the age of specialization.

My understanding of how the Brotherhood functions is, I'm sure, somewhat simplistic. I see them operating in a co-creative role with us on this planet. They design and infuse purpose and direction into the frameworks of social order through which we on Earth move in order to learn, experience and evolve. In essence, they create the schools through which we move. We call these schools religions, governmental structures, educational movements, philosophy, science . . . all those massive social frameworks with which we associate and within which we function.

My work with the Brotherhood centers around nature, of course. And the Medical Assistance Program (MAP) is an example of the Brotherhood and nature working

4

together for our benefit within an organized framework that we call MAP: The Co-Creative White Brotherhood Medical Assistance Program.

Let me tell you a little about how this program came into existence. As I have mentioned, the expansion of my work with nature into this new level of teamwork with the Brotherhood required that I physically shift and operate in new ways that would support and process the new level of work. It was such a massive jump for me that my body systems did not know how to adjust to the new demands. The first thing that occurred was that I began to misalign structurally. I had worked with a chiropractor for years previous to this as part of my general maintenance health program and I knew my body was structurally strong. I rarely needed a chiropractic adjustment. Now I needed them once or twice a month, and the adjustments were fairly extensive. At first, I said nothing to my chiropractor about the new level of work. But, after a couple of visits, she mentioned that something was odd. I was suddenly requiring a lot of adjustments and *not* requiring flower essences. (She routinely includes flower essence testing in her work.) Normally, when she sees the scope of adjustments I was needing, they are emotionally induced and require flower essence stabilization. I was not testing positive for the essences. So, questions were arising in her mind. After the second visit, during which I required as many adjustments as the first, I told her briefly what I was now doing and something about its effect on my

5

work and life. She didn't even blink. She just said that explained what she was seeing. My body didn't know how to process what I was now working with and it was "flying out of alignment" from the strain. I would need periodic adjustments while my body system was learning how to function within the new level of reality.

The second major problem I had to face was the sudden development of head pain. I felt as if my head wanted to explode. It wasn't a conventional headache— it was more like somebody had an air hose hooked up to my head and was pumping in air well beyond the capacity that my head could hold.

I returned to the chiropractor and told her about the head pressure. Luckily, she is one of the 5% of chiropractors in the United States who are trained in cranial adjustments. My physical system had to pick up the new impulses and translate them accurately in order to process what was happening to me, perceive accurately what I was working with and function well within that perception. All this is accomplished primarily within the spinal column and cranials, and it directly impacts the flow and pulsations of the cerebral spinal fluid. It is also along the spinal column that impulses are first processed by the nervous system. We could see by the adjustments I needed that all of this new action was impacting me in the spine and head. The body, not knowing both how to receive such a massive infusion of impulses *and* how to translate this input accurately, reacted by either over-loading or closing down. Physically, this would result in misalignment of vertebrae and/or misalignment or jamming of the cranials. The skull is comprised of ten major cranial bones that expand and contract according to the ebb and flow of the cerebral spinal fluid. The massive infusion of new impulses was akin to throwing a monkey wrench into the midst of all of this normal physical operation and knocking things out of kilter. Hence, the head pain.

My chiropractor and I worked together to assist my body in shifting to a different structural alignment that would better facilitate the new work I was doing. I could then learn how to process the new impulses with ease and accuracy. For a year and a half, we worked together. We responded to the glitches as they occurred (these were easy for me to detect since they resulted in various degrees of pain). The chiropractor was smart enough not to dictate what alignment I should be in; rather, she observed what alignment my body was moving towards and assisted that movement.

Our work culminated after a year and a half when my parietal cranials moved into what the chiropractor called a "parietal spread." These two massive bones at the top of the skull assumed a position allowing their expansion and contraction to operate within a new, expanded range. With this, the head pain was relieved. The chiropractor said she felt that all of our work over the past year and a half had led to this one major adjustment. We both felt that our work together had gone as far as it could go.

For a few months, all was well. But in the summer of 1984, the head pain returned. I remember I was in the

7

garden at the time when I realized that my head was beginning to hurt. I guess, as is often the case at these moments of change, I felt my work with the chiropractor was no longer feasible for practical reasons. Her office is an hour and a half driving time from Perelandra, and her practice is so large that I often had to wait a week or two for an appointment. For some reason, none of this had made any difference to me when I went to her previously. But now it was unacceptable. I felt I could not wait to have this head pain alleviated and I was now unwilling to continue driving such a long distance for what I now thought would be never-ending treatment.

I connected with the White Brotherhood, told them my problem and asked if there was something they could do to help me. They told me to go lie down, open a coning (this will be explained later) and they would connect me with help. I followed their instructions—and met Lorpuris, the head of the White Brotherhood Medical Unit.

I explained to Lorpuris what my physical discomforts were and tried to describe them as fully as I could. He instructed me to just lie quietly and comfortably, and he then set to work. The session lasted about an hour, during which I felt as if I was getting an energy charge or current through different parts of my body. It wasn't painful at all, but I must admit that it was so different from anything I had ever felt that I found the sensations to be both exciting and a little scary. At the end of the hour, Lorpuris suggested that we meet regularly so that I could go through comprehensive body balancing that would facilitate my new level of operation. I agreed and we "made a date." When I closed down the session and walked back outside, I realized that my head no longer had pain. I was amazed.

Since 1984, Lorpuris and I have continued to meet regularly. In the process of helping me physically and emotionally to adjust to my ever-expanding work and life, we explored various ways in which he and his extensive medical team could work with others here on Earth in areas of health and healing. In fact, they had been interested in making this kind of connection with us for some time.

But there were two major problems that had to be surmounted in order for us to successfully work with the White Brotherhood Medical Unit. First, there was the problem of their keying into our life system on all levels (physical, emotional, mental and spiritual) and maintaining that connection with us clearly and long enough for a medical session. We solved this problem by bringing nature on board as a member of the Brotherhood team. Now, when I connect with the medical team, I do it within a coning, a vortex of energy that includes nature intelligences, the medical team and me. Within this coning vortex, nature is able to stabilize us on all levels with the Brotherhood.

The second problem involved communication between us and the medical team. They did not want to establish a working relationship that would exclude all but the few who knew how to receive interlevel communication.

9

We solved this problem in two ways. The MAP sessions have built into them schedules and time frames that enable everyone to utilize the program even if they are unable to sense or hear anything from their team. All people have to do is follow the MAP instructions and schedule. They don't have to hear from their team when they should meet with them or for how long. This is already spelled out for them. All they have to do is talk— tell the team what is going on with them and what is out of sorts. The team can hear us effortlessly even if we can't hear them. The other solution to the communication problem was kinesiology. Those who want to ask questions and receive answers from their team can do so in a simple yes/no format. They can then "read" the answers from their team by kinesiology testing. This opens the communication door from both sides. (See Appendix A.)

Another point about communication: When we first enter the MAP program, we may not be able to hear or sense our team. (But we *will* sense things happening to us physically from time to time during the sessions.) As we continue the program, we will become used to our team, be able to better process the input from them and we will have gone through some of the clearing and adjustments necessary for us to hear and sense our team, and not just experience their work.

We have cleared up these two major stumbling blocks and, as a result, MAP was created. The shingle has been hung. The office is now open. And you are invited to enter the program.

Chapter 2

How MAP
Can Help You

To give you an idea of how MAP came into my life, I have talked about a somewhat exceptional development that most people would not encounter in their lives, but which was responsible for leading me into MAP. However, I don't want to leave the impression that MAP is only for exceptional times. It is not. MAP is for those who feel that their present medical support—whether traditional or alternative—is not enough. For years, you may feel absolutely comfortable with your medical support and then, suddenly, without a shadow of a doubt, you know you need more. To function *well* you need more input, more support. Yet, when you look around and try alternatives, none feel right. MAP is then your answer.

MAP works on your well-being from the perspective of the physical, emotional, mental and spiritual. And because of the unique position of the MAP team, it works on these levels simultaneously. Consequently, a MAP session is more comprehensive and its results are deeper than those of other health systems.

We can initiate MAP during times of illness and injury, and it can be initiated during times of relative health when we feel we are capable of a better level of health and balance—and we want it. MAP is a comprehensive health program that you will use throughout your entire life. It is not a one-time program only for emergency situations. We are constantly changing and developing throughout our lives. MAP helps us maintain a high level of balance and function throughout all our changes and shifts. In short, it gives us a chance to experience an exceptional quality of life.

We can begin MAP at any stage in our life and at any age. We do not have to be healthy to begin (some have thought this was necessary!) and we do not have to be sick. We do not need to abandon any medical support we have been using in order to begin MAP. If you are combining other health practices with MAP, this is fine. Just tell your MAP team what other things you are involved in and how. MAP will accommodate them. As I worked with my team and experienced the depth of their work, I gradually dropped, one by one, the other health practices I had been using. My confidence about MAP had to grow before I felt comfortable switching my medical needs exclusively to MAP.

It is important that you understand one thing about working with the White Brotherhood MAP team. They will not, under any circumstances, circumvent your timing on any issue. You are in complete control and command of your timing and rate of development. They will not circumvent you, because it is wrong to do so.

12

This would, in effect, remove you from the driver's seat in your own life and place you in the position of a child being catered to by the almighty parent. Your team will simply not participate in such activity.

In MAP, *you* control your timing and development in an interesting way. You will note in the instructions that you are urged to talk to your team. Tell them everything that comes to mind that is bothering you on any of your PEMS levels (physical, emotional, mental and spiritual). You aren't going through this exercise because your team is stupid and can't see you are in trouble. The troubles or situations you can articulate to your team tell them what you are ready to work on. And the extent to which you can fully describe the situation tells them the extent to which you are ready to change what is bothering you. *You are your own barometer.* They will not work in areas beyond those you recognize and describe. Consequently, your team will never put you in a position of facing and dealing with something for which you are unprepared. In the MAP session, *you* are your own master, and your team assists you in achieving your goals of health and balance in ways that are beyond belief. You are simply demonstrating your wisdom by choosing the best team with which to work.

SESSION FROM LORPURIS

I would like to add a bit to what Machaelle has already written. In short, I would like to assure you that we are eager to assist you in your quest for health and balance in any way you see fit. There will be those who will gravitate to MAP and wish to establish themselves in the MAP program, but they will hesitate because they will either feel unworthy of such an expanded approach or feel inferior, believing that we would consider it bothersome to work with them. It is this situation I would like to address.

I would like to point out that it is not a sign of good health and balance if individuals refuse help despite the fact they have gravitated towards the very help they are refusing. You might feel that I am stating the obvious. But we see the greatest stumbling block in establishing the kind of medical assistance that so many are presently seeking, either consciously or unconsciously, as being this issue of their feeling unworthy of the help. It is a vicious circle and one we cannot step in from "out of the blue" and release a person from.

*We suggest that if the concept of MAP feels right to you, yet you are feeling hesitant because you can't believe something "so good" could come to you, that you temporarily put aside your hesitancies for the purpose of entering the program. As we have said, feeling unworthy—and I use the word "unworthy" to cover feelings such as inferiority, weakness, fear and lack of capability—is a sign of being in need of help. Once you have entered the program **and have discussed with us the reasons for your hesitancies,** we will then be able to work with you to obtain a new level of balance that will effectively adjust your sense of self-worth and thus take care of the very reason you might not have entered the program.*

Since the MAP program developed as a response to my struggles with integrating an expanded level of operation, I asked Lorpuris to explain how we operate during times of expansion.

I find that people often reach the point of feeling that they need more from their medical support system because of the physical and emotional pressure that expansion experiences place on them. Expansion experiences have traditionally been relegated to spirituality, and many feel that only those who are "spiritually exulted" have expansion experiences. Well, this simply isn't true. We all have expansion experiences. Anytime we learn something new, that's expansion. Anytime we experience something new, that, too, is expansion. Whatever is new to us must be received and processed accurately and well in order for the experience to be useful.

I have said that a good sign a person needs MAP is when he has a deep sense that he needs more medical support than is presently available to him. Many feel the need for additional help when struggling with especially challenging expansion experiences because, as a rule, traditional and alternative medical systems prevalent today do not accept or understand the following: that the human body plays an essential role during expansion, how the body functions at these times and what help we need if we are not functioning well. The next session with Lorpuris will be helpful to those of you who recognize that you have been backed into a corner because of difficulties arising from expansion.

In explaining to me the role of the body in expansion, Lorpuris also gave a good explanation of how we operate as body/soul life systems on our planet. I think this will be helpful, in general, in understanding why we would feel the need for new medical assistance.

LORPURIS: HOW WE PHYSICALLY SUPPORT EXPANSION

An expanded experience does not by definition mean it to be non-physical or beyond form. It simply implies that the experience is beyond that which the person has experienced prior to that time—thus, the sense of expansion. We have said to you that the band of form is quite complex, and this is true. It includes all that a person can potentially experience while participating within any given level of form such as Earth.

While participating within a level of form such as Earth, all reality adheres to the universal law of horizontal compatibility. Consequently, what is expressed within the Earth level is "of form" whether it be discernable to the naked eye or not. The limitation regarding form arises when an individual defines form strictly from the perspective of the naked senses. Nature, for example, does not distinguish between the tree as seen by the naked eye and the nature spirit of the tree that is not seen. To nature, both are fully "of form" and, therefore, impact and respond to one another within the laws of form.

Now, the laws of form are much broader than what is encompassed when one thinks of the naked sensory system. In fact, an expanded experience is simply learning or allowing the sensory system, as most individuals know it, to operate in a fuller capacity. The problem is that individuals see the naked system as the one and only sensory system, and anything beyond or outside this base functioning as being something entirely different. In fact, they are both functions of the same system.

When a child is born into the Earth level, its sensory system is quite sensitive and expanded. It is, after all, just moving from a state of being prior to birth in which the sensory system naturally functions in a broader state. If left on its own, the child would continue to develop its sensory system from the point of this broader perspective. And what one might call "expanded experiences" would be the norm. Societal preconceptions are what encourage the child to limit the sensory scope, and the development of the sensory system throughout childhood then takes place from this more limited perspective. Along with this, the limited definition of the sensory system and its scope of discernment becomes the rule of thumb upon which to judge experience.

Now, if the sensory system is capable of naturally operating in a much broader scope than most individuals can at the present time imagine, it follows that the physical body must respond to and support that operation. The sensory system itself is a part of that overall body response and support system. Everything works as a team, ideally. Consequently, one cannot have what is known as an expanded experience without the sensory system and the physical body system as a whole responding to and attempting to support it. So, one may see a meditative state as an expanded experience, but, in fact, it is a broader use of the sensory system and calls to it appropriate response and support within the physical body itself. Just as one cannot move a finger or toe without the entire body's skeletal/muscle system responding, one cannot shift from one

17

state of mind to another without a similar physical response and shift.

There is a saying many on the Earth level use: "If you don't use it, you lose it." Normally, this refers to muscle and body tone. When a child limits the scope of operation within the sensory system, the complementary scope of physical response and support is no longer needed or utilized. In those areas, a person stiffens and atrophies. Then, later on, when the individual is an adult and consciously chooses to reactivate the sensory system in a broader way, the physical body no longer "knows" how to respond and support that expansion. The person will experience nothing, no matter how much willpower he musters, or the experience will be partially perceived and most likely distorted, as well.

Let's address the body system itself and what happens when the sensory system responds to an experience. Any experience initially strikes the human body through the electrical system. This occurs whether the experience is of the naked eye or otherwise. The initial receptor of experience is not the brain or the senses but the electrical system. The impact immediately, almost simultaneously, shifts and translates into the nervous system and routes itself throughout the nervous system appropriately as it begins its identification and experience process. This includes activating the sensory system in an appropriate manner. (All this occurs within a split second.) The point to remember is that the initial level of impact is electrical, followed by an impact in the nervous system. If the experience is within the individual's perceived notion of "acceptable," this usually means that the person knows how to perceive the experience on all levels operating within the physical body.

Two things can occur if the individual doesn't know what to do with the experience. Either the physical body doesn't know how to respond and support the experience and is in need of assistance, or the experience itself is so beyond the person's operating scope of reality that it takes on an intensification that literally overwhelms the body and requires of it a level of operation well beyond its present range of capability.

In the latter case, the person must have a good foundation for such a stretch, or else risk damaging himself physically. You would not want a person who is not capable of walking a half mile to suddenly be forced to run three miles. But you could expect that one who easily runs three miles could tackle a seven-mile run without sustaining damage. It's a challenge but not beyond the scope of possibility, and most likely not dangerous. The body, however, which is used to the exertion of the three-mile run, would have a challenge with responding well to the longer run, and it could result in soreness and discomfort until it learns to support the longer run.

Addressing the case of your 1982 expansion: You had the foundation for the challenge. You could run the three miles with ease and grace. This we were sure of. The question was how you were going to process the intensity of the new input. All that occurred was initially received within the electrical system and then shifted into the nervous system. In some ways, you responded physically much more quickly than we anticipated. In other instances, the experience overwhelmed your system and assistance was needed. Note in the work done on you by the chiropractor that she maintained close proximity to the electrical and nervous systems by concentrat-ing her work on the spine, sacrum and cranials.

Let me sum up the relationship of the cranial/spine/sacrum with the expanded experience. The experience is received electrically, shifted to the nervous system for sorting and iden-tification, and, at this point, the physical body systems move to support what is being identified. If the body cannot ade-quately shift, the electrical system will overload or break, and the corresponding vertebrae, sacrum or cranials will most like-ly react by misaligning. Hence you have the sensation of trying to catch six balls all at once while only being able to catch four.

A SPECIAL NOTE ABOUT THE CRANIALS: An expanded ex-perience carries with it an intensity that registers through the electrical system, moves into the nervous system and con-tinues its impact into the cerebral spinal fluid. The brain is impacted by both the nervous system activity and the CSF (cerebral spinal fluid) pulse response to the impact. The cranial plates must respond accordingly to accommodate this two-pronged impact. The range of plate movement will be af-fected. If the cranials have lost their knowledge of how to move within this new range or if they are three-milers stretching for the seven-mile run, they run the risk of jamming or misalign-ing. This is when so much of the head pain associated with expanded experience comes up. Cranial adjustments may be necessary over a period of time in order to allow time for the plates to properly adjust to and move in a more expanded range. One may receive these adjustments either from chiropractory or from MAP.

Just as the leg muscles need to adjust to the seven-mile run, the cranials need time to do the same. Because of the close working proximity with the electrical and nervous systems, the cranials must be considered one of the primary areas for assistance during times of expansion. In a relatively short period of time, the cranials, as well as the rest of the physical body system, will learn and will operate within the expanded range of experience with ease, accuracy and efficiency.

Chapter 3

How to Work with MAP

THE FIRST SESSION: Lie down. Get comfortable. You will need to lie on your back and remain in that position during the entire medical session. *Also, do not cross your legs or cross your hands and arms over your body.* You might wish to cover yourself with a blanket, even a thin blanket in the summer. It may make you feel more secure. If you have back pain or are having trouble getting comfortable, try placing a pillow under your knees.

1. Open the following MAP coning:
   Overlighting Deva of Healing
   Pan
   White Brotherhood: Medical Unit
   Your higher self

To open this coning, simply state:
   I would like to open a MAP coning. I would like to be connected with:
      Overlighting Deva Of Healing—Either wait 10 seconds for the connection or use kinesiology to verify the connection.

Pan—Wait 10 seconds or verify.

White Brotherhood: Medical Unit—Wait 10 seconds or verify.

My higher self—Wait 10 seconds or verify.

The coning is now open and you are ready to begin. It is not important if you did not have any sensations as the coning was activated. Your sensations or lack of sensations do not affect the quality of the coning in any way. What is important is that you be the one to call the coning into activation.

2. The first session will be for scanning purposes only. This is the one session when you need not talk if you don't wish. The purpose of this session is to key you into their level, identify your various energy patterns, lock in your life systems on all PEMS levels and get the appropriate medical team identified and working with you. Your team will work with you during all your medical sessions. Occasionally, when the situation calls for it, another doctor will join your team to lend expertise for a special situation. But your primary team will be those who work with you during the first session.

The session will last an hour. You may feel gentle shifts and energy flowing throughout your body during the session. You may even feel like you are floating or moving. You also may feel absolutely nothing. Don't worry about this. The work is going on. You might want to set a timer or alarm for 1 hour when you begin the session so that if you should drift or fall asleep, you'll know when the session is over.

At the end of the hour, request that you be given a symbol, word or sensation that you can use to identify your team. *Whatever pops into your mind next will be it.* When opening a coning for any future medical sessions, add this identification (visualize or speak it) when you call the White Brotherhood Medical Unit into the coning. This will link you more efficiently with your team. It might be good to write or draw your symbol right after this first session just to make sure you recall it accurately later on.

Your team identification can be fun. From some of the letters I've received from those who have already begun MAP, their team identification sounds like something out of the CIA code book: Torch, Lancer, Deep Rest, NIMO, Bunny-Love . . . Other people got visual symbols: the peace symbol, crosses and hands, the sun, shafts of light . . . And still others saw color. When they open the coning, they identify their team by visualizing or looking at a specific color. These identifiers don't have to be wrought with deep esoteric meaning; they just have to be something that you and your team agree upon. Also, I have heard from some folks who, after working with MAP for six months or so, wanted to change their identifying code or symbol. That's fine as long as your team is very clear about the new identification. Describe it fully to them during the MAP session. Most likely, they will either flash the new symbol or "sound" the new code word back to you to indicate their approval. Or you can kinesiology test that it is acceptable with the team.

If you do not sense a symbol or other identification code during this first session, relax. For future sessions, simply open the coning as you did the first time. You will then be connected with your team. It's like you've called into the main switchboard and then your call gets transferred to the right party. As mentioned above, using the symbol makes this process more efficient. But not using a symbol doesn't prevent your having a MAP session. Eventually, you will "receive" the symbol.

3. At the end of the hour, close the coning. You do this simply by focusing on each member of the coning separately, thanking that member, and asking to be disconnected. If you use kinesiology, verify that you are disconnected from each one by asking, "Am I disconnected?" (Test)

Spend a few moments quietly before going on about your day.

Wait 24 hours before opening the next session. The body needs 24 hours to adjust to the impact of the coning and the expansion of working with the White Brotherhood team.

REGULAR MAP SESSION PROCESS

If you use flower essences, place them within easy reach.

If you do not use flower essences or have never heard of them, I highly recommend that you investigate them and consider adding them to your health program. Having experienced MAP since 1984, I can say that flower essences are a tremendous help. Also, the MAP teams prefer you to use the essences as well. They are used in conjunction with the MAP sessions to stabilize us after the session and assist in our integrating the work the MAP team has done. There are times when the work will take, if left on its own, twenty-four hours to shift into and complete its impact on the physical body. Flower essences make these shifts efficient, effortless and complete within a two-hour period at the most. I have included information on flower essences in Appendix B. The flower essence testing instructions that are given in the steps will be understood by those who use flower essences. But again, if you do not have flower essences and don't wish to include them, this does not stop you from participating fully in MAP.

Lie down on your back. Get comfortable. Cover yourself with a blanket, if you wish.

1. Open the MAP coning:
    Overlighting Deva of Healing
    Pan
    White Brotherhood: Medical Team—Visualize your
        team's symbol or say the code word.
    Your higher self

Wait 15-20 seconds after activating the full coning so that your body can stabilize itself within the coning and with the team.

2. If they are available, test yourself for flower essences. Take the essences that you test are needed. Do not

bother getting a dosage since you will be testing again after the session is complete. If you are not using essences, skip this step.

3. Focus your attention on the session and your team. Describe *as fully as you can* how you are feeling. This includes how you feel physically, emotionally, mentally and spiritually. Relax about what you are not able to articulate. You get better with practice. *(Remember—This step is crucial for indicating your personal timing and rhythm. Your team will never alter or bypass your timing and rhythm. What you can articulate, you are ready to address.)*

4. Allow 40 minutes for the session to be completed. If you feel uncomfortable during the session, just relax and trust that at the end, whatever adjustments and shifts that are making you uncomfortable will have been completed.

If flower essences are available, ask your team during uncomfortable times if you need to test for them. Use kinesiology to get their answer. If positive, simply test the essences and take the ones you need (do not get dosage information), and then resume the session. The team will wait while you test essences.

It's important that you move around as little as possible during a session, so you will need to have the essences beside you for testing. Also, if you change your position or need to go to the bathroom during a session, tell your team to hold it a minute, do what is needed as quickly as possible, lie down again and return to the session. Sometimes their work will make you feel like you want to curl up in a fetal position. Don't do it. Just remain on your back, and shortly the team will have moved you through the process or cycle so that you will no longer feel the need to shift positions.

Another point: Don't be afraid to talk to your team during a session. It is especially helpful if you give them a running commentary of what sensations you are feeling, if any, so they can read on the spot how you are processing the work they are doing. If you suddenly feel pain, let them know where it is and how intense it is. Your body is working very hard on all of its levels to make shifts and changes. Sometimes, something gets a little "hung up" in the process. That's why your feedback is so important. (They are also open to hearing any good jokes you might have as they work.)

5. At the end of 40 minutes (add a few minutes for any essence testing or bathroom timeouts you may have taken during the session), thank your team and close the session by dismantling the coning.

Dismantling the coning is as easy as activating it. State:

> I'd like to close the coning. I'd like to disconnect from:
>> Overlighting Deva of Healing
>> Pan
>> White Brotherhood: Medical Team
>> My higher self

Wait 10-15 seconds for the dismantling to fully occur, or kinesiology test to verify that the coning is now closed.

6. Test yourself for flower essences. This time get the dosage (number of days, and number of times per day you are to take the essence solution). Begin your dosage immediately after closing down the session. You may wish to spend a few minutes quietly before continuing with your day.

NOTE: If your essence dosage period extends into your next MAP session, discontinue that dosage after this session and test for new essences and a new dosage. Each MAP session will wipe the essence slate clean and will begin a new solution of essences and dosage.

MAP Session Schedule

First month: twice weekly

Second through fourth months: once weekly

Fifth month and on: twice monthly (For balancing and general maintenance.)

During times of difficulty, illness or while going through periods of expansion: twice weekly. If you sense more is needed: 3-4 times weekly.

Once you can communicate with your team, either through kinesiology or intuitive input, you can ask for specific guidelines for the scheduling that is geared to you personally.

A SUGGESTION: The Brotherhood has put together this "beginner's schedule" that covers a period up to five months. When deciding if you would like to participate in the program, I suggest that you make a five-month commitment to MAP—and then decide after the five months if you want to *continue* participating in the program. There are many things I can say about MAP and my experiences with it. But, to be honest, I can't adequately express to you in words how different and phenomenal this program is. You have to experience it for yourself. And, to appreciate what the program can do for you, you have to experience it for more than one or two sessions. After five months, you will have gone through all of the timing sequences and established yourself in the twice-a-month rhythm. I feel at this point you will be able to make a good decision. And, by this time, you will see that you really can integrate MAP into your life without causing a major upheaval to your schedule.

ANOTHER SUGGESTION: Keep notes on the sessions. Record the difficulties and problems you talked about, sensations you felt during the sessions and results you perceived after the session. At some point down the road, these notes often reveal patterns in us we had no idea existed. They also help confirm to *ourselves* that something really is happening in MAP. It's not our imagination. And, sometimes, we go into a period of the MAP work when we feel *nothing*. We swear nothing is happening. We even entertain the notion that perhaps our team has walked out on us! But, it's just that the work they are doing is, for the time being, on levels we can't perceive. We'll come out of this period and once again feel things during the sessions. In the meantime, a casual review of the notes reminds us that, indeed, these sessions are for real.

Chapter 4

What Happens in a MAP Session

I have worked with MAP since the summer of 1984 and have gone through many different schedules with the team ranging from daily sessions to once a week or every three days. I have always allowed them to set a suggested pace, feeling that I would receive more from MAP if I listened to my team. The scheduling did not correspond with specific physical or emotional "rough periods" when one might expect an increased need for MAP. Instead, they seemed to increase my schedule when my life became intense and it was imperative that my balance be maintained throughout.

What I would like to relate to you now is not only some of my experiences, but also suggestions based on my experiences and my work around MAP with Lorpuris.

The sessions are always different. I can never count on a session to be one way or another, even after all this time. When *I* think something is happening in my life that warrants a difficult session, I may get a gentle, easy one. I often have tough sessions when I least expect them. If I enter a session with a complaint about my right shoulder being stiff, I may feel them working on my left foot throughout the session. After the session, my right shoulder feels fine.

During the easy sessions I can feel absolutely nothing. I know I am connected with my team and we may be "chatting" back and forth, but I can't feel them working on me. (I have accused them of gold-bricking!) At other times, I will feel my body gently move. I even feel that I'm being turned over or that I'm floating. Of course, when I look at myself, I'm still on the bed. But had I not opened my eyes, I would never have guessed that I had not physically moved. Sometimes I feel "electrical currents" flowing throughout my body or through part of my body. Sometimes I feel tingling sensations. All these things are quite pleasant.

During the tough sessions, I feel pain. Sometimes—but not often—it's difficult pain. Usually the pain centered around emotional releases, and I have learned that emotional pain is truly as physically tangible as physical pain. When the pain comes, I tell my team. Then I ask if I should test for essences. Sometimes they say yes, sometimes they say it's not necessary. (This is where kinesiology testing comes in handy for you.) As intense as the pain may get, my team has *always* brought me full circle by the end of the session and the pain is no longer present. I have never left a session with the pain. One of my suggestions to you, that I practice constantly, is to tell your team when pain occurs, how intense it is and where it is located. I also tell them when the intensity either increases or decreases.

A fun reaction when I have dealt with emotions has been the sensation that little "champagne bubbles" of energy bubble up through my chest and just pop out. This often makes me laugh.

Sometimes I'll be "bopping along" in my session and, all of a sudden, I'll start spontaneous deep breathing that will go on for some minutes. And then just as suddenly, I'll stop breathing deeply. During these times, I will relax and go with the impulses.

At other times, I cry. The odd thing is that it seems as if the team has hit a "cry button" and I just start crying. Sometimes I feel the specifics of the emotion, sometimes not. Sometimes insights surface, sometimes not. I also have had insights after the session when I was just going about my day again. Something comes to mind out of the blue, and everything from the session falls into place.

Most of the time after a session, I feel fine. I have never been "left hanging" by my team. They seem to work in a rhythm that completes itself within the context of a single session. Sometimes I feel tired after a session, but a nap or a night's sleep takes care of that. Also, I usually feel vulnerable about the session itself, and I choose not to talk to anyone about the specifics. I feel very close to my team and focus our work solely with them.

A handful of times over these past years, I have been

absolutely fine after a session, and then the next day I take on a sudden, unexplainable pain that seems to come from nowhere. I have learned that at these times my body's adjustment to the work done has hit a glitch. As soon as I can, I will open a MAP session and tell them what is going on. Each time they have taken care of the problem.

Being a part-time klutz, I am sometimes prone to an accident or two. I work extensively with flower essences, so when I have an accident, I immediately check myself for essences. Then I open a MAP session and tell them what I have done to myself—this time. They have neutralized wasp stings, completely eliminated a black eye (I had hit my eye on a hook and it was well on its way to being a nasty black eye in about 15 minutes.) and worked me through a severely sprained ankle to the point that I was walking without a limp in two days. They are also whiz-bangs at getting rid of sinus headaches.

I don't ask them a lot of questions about what they are doing. I know there are some who are using MAP and just need to know everything. Oftentimes these people are not yet capable of communicating directly with their team and become frustrated about not knowing exactly what is going on. Quite frankly, I don't want to know all the nuts and bolts about what my team is doing. I sense that they are working in ways that I, at best, would barely understand. Instead, I focus on how I am reacting and responding to their work—and on the results of MAP. This way, I learn more about myself, recognize what I am experiencing from MAP and am more capable of giving my team the quality feedback they need about how I am functioning. In short, I let my MAP team do their job and I do mine.

When I first talked about MAP at a workshop, I cautioned people not to open a session if they are tired and likely to fall asleep. I still say this but, based on the letters I got back, I need to modify it a little. It is important that, whenever possible, you not come into a session in such an exhausted state that you konk out in the first five minutes. However, just about everyone who was working with MAP reported that they often fell asleep in the sessions no matter what they did. I asked Lorpuris about this and he said that the team will put you in a sleep state at certain times when it is important for the work being done. Usually, an especially mentally active person who is getting "in the way" of the work will be put in a sleep state. When they need you to be alert, they will wake you up again. So, *your* responsibility will be to enter the MAP session when you can maintain alertness and interact with your team. However, if you find you are going to sleep anyway, just relax about it. You have done your part by intending to be awake as you move through the session.

By the way, the 40-minute time for a session begins *after* the coning has been opened and you have checked yourself for flower essences.

If there are other people in your family who decide to work with MAP, your session schedules will not conflict with one another. You can all have your MAP sessions at the same time. MAP isn't a doctor's office where everyone has to wait his turn. However, if more than one MAP session is going on in the house simultaneously, make sure you are not all in the same room. Each person needs to be in his own room.

Sometimes people wake up during the night and feel they need a session. You can have a session in bed next to your spouse or partner *if* you can get at least a 3-foot clear space between you. Your team will have difficulty with the impact of another energy field from this person if he or she—or the dog— is too close. If you don't have enough clear space, I'm afraid you'll have to go into another room for the session.

If the flu or any such illness is running through the family and you don't yet have it, nor do you want it, have frequent MAP sessions throughout the siege. Your team will help you maintain your balance and keep up your strength.

I have not needed surgery or broken any bones; consequently, I have not worked with MAP with these situations. But in discussing this with Lorpuris, I feel I would let common sense prevail and have conventional surgery or a broken bone set—and then have MAP assist me during recovery. In short, I'd utilize the best medical practices possible for exceptional needs requiring quick physical attention. At the same time, I'd look to MAP for assistance in any preparation I might require and the more complex areas of repair and healing resulting from the injury or surgery.

MAP SESSIONS FOR CHILDREN

Generally, children do not need the kind of intensive help that MAP offers and there are other means that can be utilized to get comprehensive help for them. For example, flower essences. This is a simple, efficient and *extremely* effective tool for balancing and helping children. And it is something they can relate to and enjoy taking. Flower essences are not a mystery to them—they can see, feel, smell and taste the essences. MAP sessions may be scary since the child will be sensing and feeling things he or she won't be able to relate to or understand.

If you absolutely feel that your child needs MAP, you must be prepared to function as his or her support throughout the entire session. My first suggestion is that you do not attempt to activate MAP for a child until you have worked with MAP yourself for *at least five months.* As I said, you will need to remain with a child for the entire session and assist him or her throughout. This means that you will need to surrogate test and administer the flower essences to the child. You will also have to know enough about the different sensations to be able to assure the child if he or she becomes frightened. And you will need to be able to communicate directly with the MAP team, either using kinesiology or whatever other method you have developed, in order to discern specifics that the team wishes to pass along as well as the child's session schedule. The MAP team will not put a child in a lengthy series, but rather will consider its work with the child to be due to special situations requiring a shorter schedule. In essence, you have to be confident enough about MAP to function as a competent, relaxed support person. Under no circumstances do I recommend that you activate MAP for a child unless you can meet these criteria.

I also would like to point out that you should not activate MAP for a child unless you are the legal guardian of the child or have permission from that child's legal guardian. I don't mean to emphasize law here, but rather intent. Legal guardianship implies certain rights between an adult and a child that include the right to make this kind of decision for the child.

If you feel a child must have MAP, *you* will activate the coning for the initial scanning session. You must include both your higher self *and* the child's higher self in the coning. You will need to inform the Brotherhood that you are acting on behalf of a child. Allow 10-15 seconds to pass for them to adjust the coning appropriately in order to facilitate what you want. (The child can be asleep for the scanning session and all regular sessions. You may prefer this since it is easier to keep a sleeping child still! If possible, it would be best for the child to be lying on his or her back. But if this is not possible, the team will work around it.) Then, placing your two hands side by side, palms down and parallel to the reclining child without touching the body, "scan" the child's body system to the team. This differentiates your body energy from the child's. Do this by moving your hands in concert, starting from the top of the head and moving slowly down the body to the bottoms of the feet. As you move down the trunk, you will have to scan each arm and then each leg. The movement of your hands should be slow and steady. If you can "hear" the team, they may tell you to hold the scanning at certain spots along the way. Just stop your hands and hold them above the body until you get the go-ahead to start the scan again. The first session will last an hour. At the end, *you* will receive the child's team symbol or code. Close down the session exactly as you would for yourself, only now you must disconnect from your higher self *and* the child's higher self. Also, test the child for essences (see the book, *Flower Essences*, for surrogate testing steps), and check yourself for essences, just in case your being in this special coning threw your balance off.

The regular session conings are activated in the same manner as for yourself, except you will use the child's symbol or code instead of yours and include the child's higher self. It is important that you not hold the child during the session because the mixing of the two sets of energy will be too much for the team to separate and discern well. However, if you must touch the child for essence testing during the session or hold the child if he or she should become frightened, you may do so. The team will stop the session until you are finished. The regular sessions for a child are also 40 minutes. Find out from the team when they wish to work with the child again. It won't be like the adult schedule. Close down the coning and check both you and the child for flower essences and solution dosages.

MAP EXPERIENCES BY OTHERS

In 1989, I introduced MAP during a workshop. The folks were given the steps and encouraged to try the program. Several months later, I sent out a letter asking them for feedback as to whether they were working with MAP and what their experiences were. Out of 50 workshop participants, 30 responded that they were now working with MAP. They gave me permission to use portions of their letters so that others could benefit from their experiences and thoughts. And I felt it would be good for you to know that others besides myself are benefitting from MAP.

The following are excerpts from their letters. I have chosen letters that would show you both the similar patterns these people experienced with MAP and some of their different experiences.

> . . . I was not ready to do this kind of work for a long time. I respected that as an indication that the timing wasn't right for me yet. I also think I wasn't yet ready to make the commitment to go through whatever changes would be involved. However, during the past holidays, I began to feel that the time was right to begin. So, after checking with my higher self to make sure, I had my first session in January.

My scanning session seemed fairly uneventful. I had the sense nothing was happening yet, other than everybody getting acquainted. I did get my symbol when I asked. An image of a torch popped into my head as soon as I asked.

I have been doing the sessions twice weekly, but have just gone to a once-weekly schedule. My normal time to do them is about 8:00 P.M. I start by making the coning connection as you outlined. Then I ask if I need any essences and take them. I keep a notebook handy and record the essences and any issues and experiences that come out of the session. I do the sessions in bed, usually with a pillow under my legs . . . I set a timer in the kitchen for 45 minutes, and then go into the bedroom. By the time I connect, test for essences and get into bed, about 40 minutes are left for the session. Usually, I sense that the session is winding down a few minutes before the timer goes off. I thank everybody, close the coning and retest for essences.

I have felt very little physically while in the sessions, including the initial scanning session. There has been no pain or unpleasantness so far, except for one session where I felt very restless and found it hard to be still.

I think the main issue we've been working

on has been an emotional one, centered around my self-worth. Often, I start the session drifting off into sleep, only to awaken suddenly with some image or flash of insight, and a sense of clarity and light about who I am and what I'm doing here in this present life. It seems like maybe the drifting off is the way we have of getting my day-to-day mind out of the picture for a while so that the rest of my mind can say something to me. I do feel that the insights are coming from me, and that MAP is just facilitating the process.

I have had a couple of more physical experiences. Once, I felt embraced by a very warm and loving being, in an aura of total acceptance. It was an immediate kind of thing, not something airy-fairy. Another time, I felt like I was filled by a clear, bright light that made me buoyant. Both of these only lasted for seconds, but were so strong that the feelings lingered way past the session, and are actually there whenever I remember them.

It took me a couple of sessions to get used to doing it, but now I make a point of verbalizing what issues I'm bringing into the sessions and what I'm experiencing during it . . . Speaking makes things clearer to everyone involved.

The main word I have for how the MAP team works with me is "unobtrusive." I know they're there and I feel things happening, but it's subtle. It's like they take their cues from me and never force anything. The image I have is that exercise where two people face each other and one makes movements that the other duplicates, so that the first person feels like he's looking at his image in a mirror. It's that quality I feel from the team. They're that sensitive.

After almost two months of sessions, I have to say that MAP is very helpful and really pretty easy to do, once you make the commitment to do it. I have felt more clarity in my life and a greater sense of being connected with a larger reality. I credit MAP for some of the moves I'm making in my Feldenkrais work. I've found that MAP doesn't eliminate any issues or any work on my part but makes it all flow better. I have this image of the team squirting all the creaky, rusty joints of my being with oil to make them work smoothly . . . C.W., Virginia

. . . Yes, I have been using MAP; and, yes, it is a test of faith. I waited until November 8 to begin, because I needed to address lingering issues of self-worth first—i.e., the belief that my life and work are not "important" enough in the universal scheme of things to "deserve" such specialized medical treatment. I knew from the moment they began surfacing that these thoughts were/are erroneous, but the more deeply-anchored feelings accompanying them kept me from contacting the WB Medical Team and requesting their services. Working through these feelings eventually led me to realize the significance of the law of free will and also Jesus' statement "Ask and you shall receive." . . . K.W., Michigan

. . . My basic issue centers around feeling comfortable with something that is beyond my five senses. I have experienced subtle body sensations, seen energy patterns swirling in front of my eyes and gotten hunches that I should do things, but I still sometimes get angry at myself that I don't experience these sessions with greater conscious awareness.

Interestingly enough, in spite of not feeling competent about my ability to sense what's going on, the initial scanning session seemed very real to me. I needed essences to start the session. I got my team's name easily . . . I saw something which I interpreted as my team's symbol (a swirling circle of energy which was also pulsating and contained a number of brilliant points of light or stars). I also felt some tingling in my arms and legs as if energy were being run through them . . . C.P., Virginia

. . . After I attended your workshop, I knew immediately that I had to work with MAP. The problem that I have hasn't been helped in 12 years with medical practice. The scanning session went well. I felt energy going up my spine and head area. At times I felt back pain, neck pain and uncomfortable. I received no symbol.

During my first session, I spaced out several times. They were spinning my head around (a very strange experience!), worked on the cranium and especially on the right side of the head. Also spun my hands around and worked on the hands. Then I was given a symbol.

Oddly enough, in the beginning I bought a little notebook and recorded everything in it. I usually don't take notes or record. But alas, it came in handy.

I have no fear about this work, but then I perceive mostly through intuition. Sometimes I feel like an idiot lying there for 40 minutes talking to the air. At that point I'll say, "Please give me a sign you are there. I feel so dumb." And then I would feel someone brushing against my forehead or hair. Without doubt, I know that someone is there with me . . . R.S., Pennsylvania

. . . Scanning session: I was very excited and curious to start the process . . . I felt a little awkward not knowing who or what I was talking to. I felt the presence of four—three males and one female. I asked if that was correct and received an affirmative. For most of the first session I just listened and "felt" what was happening. I did feel a lot of movement, pressure, all around me, especially around my head and abdomen. I would occasionally describe what I was feeling and ask if it was them. I would always receive an affirmative reply by "testing." The interesting thing to me is I have felt the same "kinds" of sensations almost nightly for as long as I can remember—pressures around my head, in my temples, in the roof of my mouth, etc. I don't know if there is any connection. When I try to question in that area, the answers are a little "fuzzy."

For the rest of the sessions, meaning up until now, I haven't perceived the presence of anyone but continue to feel the energy sensations—although at times it is so subtle that I sometimes wonder if it is all my imagination. Close to the end of the first month, I started asking for some kind of confirmation. That is when I started "dreaming" a *lot* . . .

The only consistent part of the sessions has been that no matter how hard I try, or the time of day or night of the sessions, *I always fall asleep* if for only the last few minutes. Then I will wake up only to find the session over.

I have had several dreams of a more direct nature—dreams where rooms or houses were being remodeled, etc. They seem more clearly recognizable . . .

Re: how I have felt changes. I have felt I have some unseen helpers that I can call on during times of mental or emotional stress and have done so with subtle but positive results in smoothing over rough spots. I "feel" that I am in some kind of "process" that I can't really articulate, but I feel comfortable and good about it. I feel a seriousness about the process—don't know if it's me reflecting back to me or if I am actually perceiving the team to be a really serious team. A little kidding around would be welcome—I think . . . J.B., Virginia

. . . Even though I was thrilled to receive the MAP technique at the workshop, it took me 2 or 3 weeks to get up enough nerve to start doing it.

The scanning session was interesting. I felt like I was being scanned by different energy sources in a very methodical way—from top to bottom and sideways. In my mind's eye, I "saw" different colors as the different scans were done. I also had impressions of different large instruments being pointed at me. One was something like the projector used in a planetarium, sort of. My symbol is the sun . . .

My first session was quite unsettling. My father died in October after a long decline. What they had me do was deep breathing, then I became very nauseated and almost threw up, then I started to shout, "I hate my father." In fact, for the next week, I periodically said that, either in my head or out loud. During the whole time, I felt detached and kept thinking, "Isn't this interesting?" During the second session, I also did deep breathing to the point where I thought I was going to go into a re-birthing experience, but I didn't. Subsequent sessions have been much gentler at my request . . .

Since June I have been trying to get over thyroiditis, mainly working with my chiropractor to rebuild my immune system. I also practice the Radiance Technique . . . I give myself a treatment every morning in bed before I get up. When I told my team about the Radiance, they said to set up the coning and give myself my treatment, and they would work "within the energy." So for about three to four weeks now I've been doing that. I also experimented doing it without MAP after a week to see if I could tell the difference, and I really can. The energy is really amplified . . . I don't talk out loud to them, only in my head. I don't "see" them physically or in my mind's eye, only feel their energy and sometimes, at the end of my treatment, I am filled with golden light and warmth and am surprised to see that the sun is not shining when I open my physical eyes . . . M.L., Virginia

. . . Scanning session: Felt light and floating most of the time. Sensation of energy around me and a bright light. Received symbol of "cactus." Now, when this first came to me, I immediately questioned it. I said to myself, "What? A cactus?" Then I just said, "accept it" and went on. The whole experience was very subtle, nothing dramatic.

Second session: During the day (before I did the second session) I felt very spacey, could not concentrate. I had pain in my stomach and abdominal area—seemed to be in the muscles running up and down and across my whole area. This sounds odd, but I had the feeling that my body, soul and heart had regrouped, had pulled together. As if before, I had been sort of spread out and when I walked around I was dragging and catching on things. Now, I felt compact, strong and more gathered in.

The pain cleared up about 30 minutes before I did the second session. After the session, I felt exhausted. It was hard to make notes and test for essences again. During the session I had no trouble talking with my team. I felt energy going through me again and again. I felt pain in my shoulders and back during the physical discussion. I had to swallow a lot and it seems like I was told to do that. I slept very deeply afterwards.

Third session: Was a very bright, positive session. Lots of energy, feeling of weightlessness very pronounced . . . S.D., Pennsylvania

. . . I started using MAP within a week of the workshop. Since I use the Energy Cleansing Process, I was comfortable in invoking the four participants in the energy coning. I'm not a little awed and humbled at the generosity of the Deva of Healing, Pan, the WB Medical Unit and even my Higher Self, in making themselves so readily available . . .

I find it easy to talk with them and joke with them. For example, while I picture that they are working on me to help me physically accommodate spiritual expansion, I tell them that helping me relieve myself of some cellulite around my thighs would also be very welcome. I tell them about emotional issues I'm working on, e.g., resentment, aches and pains I've got, e.g., chronic tight sore throat, aching joints, how my eyesight is changing rapidly, what events are going on in my life (e.g., my kids both have a bad case of chicken pox, my spouse is living across the continent with no plans for returning). I feel energy moving in my body during the sessions, particularly at the base of the spine and up my spinal cord. I also feel sensations in my neck, head, shoulders, pelvis and the bottoms of my feet. It seems to me so far that the more I give them immediate feedback as to what I'm feeling, the faster the next sensations come. It's been pretty amazing, but never overwhelming. Frequently, I am relieved of aches and pains I had when I first lay down.

The biggest "problem" I have is finding the privacy and time for the sessions. (I'm essentially a single parent of an infant and a kindergartener and I work and I'm 41 years old. Age gives me an edge on wisdom perhaps, but physically the child-rearing is harder.) I have even gotten a babysitter to have sessions . . .

What I feel overall from the sessions is that they are fine-tuning me physically and energetically and I have an increased general sense of well-being. I feel emotionally nurtured from the sessions. And it seems they work very well with the other healing and spiritual work I am doing.

. . . I've had a few sessions unlike the others. During the first two of the unusual sessions, I fell asleep—it was irresistible and I felt that it was OK with my WB team. I was jolted awake (a big *soft* jolt) with a flash of white light in my chest. I pictured the team with the energy equivalent of one of those heart machines that are used to shock people's hearts into restarting. I dozed off again and got zapped again. It was a surprising sensation, but not unpleasant.

The third session I want to tell you about felt like a non-event by contrast, at least initially. I wasn't aware of any sensations, energy moving, etc., as usual. I considered that I wasn't having a MAP session. As I lay there though, I realized that what I was labeling as "mental drifting" was much more vivid and meaningful than that. It felt like I was getting a lesson from my unconscious or right brain, and the pictures were in fact helping me to understand the issue I had asked my team to address at the beginning of the session. I don't know if the MAP works that way (through pictures, insights, awake dreams) or not, but I feel I was getting some extra help from somewhere . . . B.G., Florida

. . . I find the sessions very enjoyable. The particular quality of awareness that comes during the sessions is unique in my experience. It is akin to certain experiences I've had from meditating and other practices, but has a distinct quality of its own. I usually feel a particular sense of expansion and peace that is wonderful and have found that the peace extends into my daily life more and more. This peace pervades the session—particularly during the first part of it. Even though I feel quite a few physical sensations during the sessions, some of them unpleasant, at the same time I feel quite detached from them. Toward the latter part of the session I often feel more "in the body" and the sensations are not as comfortable. I occasionally feel worse physically at the very end of the session but have found that the discomfort passes quickly once I become active. . . .

I have made very specific requests as to what I want from the sessions and I have to say that these requests are being granted in a way that borders on the miraculous. I started out with some pretty major imbalances and am feeling that balance is coming quickly and profoundly. I started the Garden and Rose Essences a few weeks before I began the healing sessions and found that they started to help . . . and then these benefits accelerated dramatically once I began the MAP sessions. The combination has been extremely beneficial—bringing greater health, clarity, functionality and peace of mind. . . . M.K., Virginia

WHAT DOES NOT HAPPEN IN A MAP SESSION

You are in control of the coning at all times. The MAP teams do not open a coning on their own. You must do this. And the teams will not refuse to close down a coning. Once you indicate a coning is to be closed, it is closed. The teams will not ignore or override your requests. Also, your coning is perfectly protected. Nothing more needs to be done to "shore it up." However, someone who has paranoia tendencies or extreme victimization problems should not enter into the MAP program. They will not be able to accurately discern what is happening to them and will automatically turn MAP into a frightening experience. If such a thing is happening to you, stop using MAP immediately and work on your personal issues in ways that don't set up an automatic fear response. No matter what, MAP cannot protect you from yourself.

MAP will not solve your business problems or get involved in local government issues. It is a *medical* program. It is also a *human* medical program. MAP is not intended for animal care. (See p. 128 listing of Perelandra Paper #8: *Nature Healing Conings for Animals*.)

They will not leave you dangling. They do not do more than can be completed in forty minutes.

The MAP teams are not hoodlums. They do not kill your plants or steal your money. (Don't laugh—a couple of people accused their teams of such activity.) Although you will experience love and respect from your team, they will not say things like you are the only one who can save the world—then proceed to give you a long list of wacky things to do for saving said world. These are all self-conjured experiences that spring out of fear or a deep desire to "live a significant life." If you are having such experiences or are "hearing voices" that say strange things and won't stop, tell your team and let them help you regain your balance.

Chapter 5

The Calibration Process

In early 1990, nature came up with a brilliant process that is designed to balance us during times of emotional and mental stress through which we have difficulty moving. I immediately began working with this process and found that the Calibration Process can be easily combined with the MAP session.

First, let me introduce the Calibration Process to you as it was given to me in a nature session. Included are my comments about working with the process. Then I'll explain why it can and should be added to MAP and how.

SOME PERSONAL COMMENTS
ON THE CALIBRATION PROCESS

I have worked with this process extensively since I translated the Calibration Process session in March 1990. I wanted to understand and experience it before offering it to others, and I wanted to explore the different ways in which the process could be used. From the very first time I worked with it, I was amazed. I'd like to pass along to you some of my feelings about the process and give you ideas about when it can be used.

What impressed me first was the efficiency of the Calibration Process. It only takes a half-hour once you've explained the problem. Initially, I questioned this, not believing that so little time was needed to accomplish so much. In all of my work with the Calibration Process, the sessions have not exceeded the time it takes to express the problem and the half-hour. I'm quite used to nature coming up with exceptional co-creative processes that redefine the concepts of efficiency and effectiveness, but I was still impressed this time around.

It took a little thinking on my part to figure out when I was in a situation that could be helped by the Calibration Process. It is *not* needed if we are moving through an emotional or mental process where we have a sense of forward motion being maintained. It's useful when we feel our wheels spinning or feel stuck and can't even begin to imagine how we are to proceed—we're at a dead end. The Calibration Process doesn't sidestep us from emotional and mental processes. It is designed to keep our processes moving on all of our levels and "unjam" those places where we seem to have gotten stuck.

The first time I used the process in March 1990, I knew I was having difficulty addressing my work in the garden and maintaining focus on what I needed to do. I had tried every trick I knew that I thought might "wake me up." I might feel my ability to focus return, but it would be short-lived and I would quickly sink into what felt like a hole. I decided to try the Calibration Process. I set it up exactly as it is written in the session. I tried to explain as simply and succinctly as possible how I was feeling and how my life was being affected. And I admitted that I knew nothing else I could try. I sat for the half-hour and felt nothing happening. I closed the coning as instructed, assuming something would occur that would tip me off that I was now "healed" or whatever. Since I had done this session in the evening, I went about my "off hours" as usual. I still noticed nothing different by the time I went to bed. The next day, I began my day without thinking about either the process or possible changes. I just got on with what I had wanted to do. By the end of the day, it occurred to me that not only had I accomplished everything I could have hoped to do and more, but I had done all of this effortlessly. Not once did I feel I had to deliberately press myself through a project. I simply did it.

I wanted to share this first experience with you because it shows so clearly how the process can work without a bunch of bells and bugles sounding. In this instance, one day I was in one state of being (a difficult, unconstructive, wheel-spinning state) and the next day, after doing the process, I was in a completely different state of being. I didn't experience a linear progression from the first state to the next. I simply found myself in it. Sometimes I have found in this process that there aren't any great moments of understanding and resolution. At times I have felt that the gears between my emotional and mental levels and my body are simply "off" and in need of a little calibration. So, nature gets everything back into sync, and the dams that seem to cause the wheel-spinning unjam, and that's all it takes.

At other times, I did go through a resolution and understanding process that occurred either within the half-hour or within the twenty-four hours after the process. Again, it wasn't like some baseball bat hitting me in the head. Nothing that dramatic. I'd be moving along in my day and suddenly I'd know what the troublesome issue really was. Usually that in itself was the resolution. Or sometimes the resolution was in the form of action I needed to take to complete the issue.

I have used the Calibration Process when I was mentally buzzing and couldn't stop, when I couldn't stop working and when I could see that a fear I was experiencing was actually counter-productive and not helpful. Or, for some crazy reason, I found myself unable to make a decision even when I had all the information and input I needed. Another example: When I began the annual workshop series this year at Perelandra, I worked with the Calibration Process to shift me from my predominant role as the researcher to add the dynamic of the teacher. I found myself approaching and setting up the workshops in ways I had not even considered before—and it was better.

Everything I have experienced from this process verifies to me what nature says about the need to strike an involution/evolution balance within ourselves in order to function well. All my experiences have been accurate, efficient and effective. In working with the process, I have grown and developed around the area of emotional/mental balance in ways that allow me to more clearly see new areas where this process could be useful. If I suspect a Calibration Process would be helpful, I'll open the Healing Coning and ask:

Is this a situation that could be helped with the Calibration Process?

So far, I've always been told yes.

UNDERSTANDING THE ISSUES HUMANS FACE AND WHY IT IS IMPERATIVE TO LINK IN CONSCIOUS PARTNERSHIPS WITH NATURE

It is becoming increasingly important for humans to understand the extensive partnership they have with nature, especially when focusing on issues of form and energy and all that this combination implies. We are presently in an interesting time in human development that has not been prevalent to this great extent at any other time. We refer to the fact that the desires and needs of the human soul on Earth completely outstrip the ability of the present support frameworks. By this we mean support frameworks in all areas: agricultural, scientific, physical health, mental and emotional health, governmental, social, educational . . . The development of the human soul collectively on Earth has surpassed the development of its support systems. In a nature-dominant environment that existed on the planet until the last fifty or so years, the human soul could more easily develop support systems that were compatible. One reason for this is that nature was abundant and could accommodate every human's needs. (We do not mean to imply that all needs were met, only that all needs could have been met had humans so chosen.) The physical means for all human support could have been met at any time because of natural abundance.

In the past fifty years, this balance has shifted and the planet has become human-dominant. Nature is no longer abundant enough to accommodate human needs and desires without careful consideration regarding the larger picture. We do not see this as a "bad" development. If ignored, however, it will be a dangerous development for all. But it is also a development that is forcing the human soul to expand on every level in order to address and survive the severe challenges that the shift to a human-dominant planet has created. Prior to this shift, individual human souls could expand and develop in ways that were not associated with survival. In short, there was a sense of leisure around the kind of expansion of which we speak. The individual had a lifetime to expand his understanding of life from a broader perspective while, at the same time, he devoted his efforts and energy primarily into those activities that served to support his day-to-day physical survival. Now, for the sake of survival on all levels, the human soul is required to make this shift, this expansion, and to do it quickly.

The present support systems were designed to best address human survival in a nature-dominant era that simultaneously existed within a Piscean context (parent/child emphasis). You are now seeing the shift to a human-dominant era that is simultaneously being impacted by the Aquarian impulses (partnership, balance and teamwork emphasis). All of the previously workable support systems are crumbling. At the same *time, humans are expanding. By this we mean that the human in the conscious state is expanding to enfold the human spirit in the unconscious state. With this fusion, when it occurs, the unconscious becomes conscious. Humans are beginning to understand in an immediate and personal way that life is far broader and more complex than they ever before understood. This expansion does not occur in a vacuum. It requires support on all PEMS levels (physical, emotional, mental, spiritual) in order for it to be stabilized and maintained. So you have humans expanding in their efforts to address serious survival issues on all levels while, at the same time, having to function within a collection of frameworks that were never designed to meet the pressures of the present issues. There is an ever-expanding gap between today's expanding human and the planet's various social support systems' capabilities.*

We have not gone off the topic of presenting the co-creative Calibration Process. We are giving you the background needed to understand the crux of the issues that humans face as well as why it is now so imperative for them to link in conscious partnerships with nature in order to develop the support systems of the future—and we mean by this the near-future!

The expansion of the human system requires that the expertise of nature in the areas of the relationship of form to energy and involution (bringing spirit and purpose into form) be tapped in direct proportion to the expansion. In your vernacular, the intensity and complexity of the game have increased to such a degree that the relative simplicity of the old support systems has been rendered ineffective. Humans must partner with nature in order to establish the systems that will support the new complexity. Don't forget—the expansion of the human consciousness to enfold its unconsciousness includes the grounding of the entire expansion into form. Otherwise, the expansion will either falter or take on an ungrounded air and be useless. This expansion process is what is referred to as "the evolution dynamic." The grounding of the expansion and its expression through form is what is meant by "the involution dynamic." The human soul is being pressed to open beyond or soar above the existing support systems on the planet in order to see the new. To properly support this expansion, the development of systems enfolding the balance between the involution dynamic and the evolution dynamic is imperative.

And this is what nature can give you now. It understands the relationship of energy to form and it knows what is required in order for spirit and the soul's direction and purpose to perfectly seat into form in balance. As we have pointed out a number of times, nature is the master of involution and the expert in matters involving the relationship of energy to form. In order to create support systems that respond to this new demand of human souls seeking to ground a broader picture of reality into form, man must turn to nature.

We do not mean to imply that if man turns to nature for the needed development of his support systems that this development will be effortless and perceived as perfect. We have no intention of perpetuating a parent/child dynamic in our relationship with mankind. We have no intention of dictating structure and process. In fact, this would be impossible. Humans must supply intent, purpose, direction and need when it comes to systems development. With this definition, we in nature will seek to supply the best structure in which to accommodate and move intent, purpose, direction and need. It is a true partnership we seek. We will not interfere with or attempt to alter the human evolutionary thrust. We are here to assist and accommodate this thrust.

In medicine, humans have seen the relationship of nature to themselves in the areas of nutrition, natural medicines and stress relief. Humans do not see themselves as nature/human soul systems requiring involution/evolution balance. Instead, they see themselves as souls utilizing nature in form for the purpose of evolutionary growth. Nature has been the servant of the soul while the primary thrust of the human has been evolutionary. This cannot and does not work. The human system itself is a partnership between soul and nature, and its thrust, its primary focus, is the involution/evolution balance. When in form, and we mean by this any existence within the band of form, the human must strive for involution/evolution balance in order to achieve evolutionary movement. Without this balance, there is no evolutionary movement, activation or change. The involution dynamic is the tool of the movement, activation and changes required by the evolution dynamic.

THE ARENA OF EMOTIONAL/MENTAL HEALTH

First of all, let us say that we refer to this arena as "emotional/mental" because the dynamics causing a person to be classified in need of emotional or mental assistance are, from nature's perspective, the same. The distinction between the two is created by humans and does not concern nature.

You will recall, Machaelle, from your personal exploration in this area that when you came upon an emotional block that seemed impossible for you to get through, you asked us in nature for help. We will say now that the insight to ask for help was, in fact, initiated from us of nature and in response to our desire to assist you in any way possible. You picked up on this insight and acted on it by opening with the intent for us to assist you. It is essential that people understand that in areas where nature links with the human soul, it (nature) can only do so on request. We do not assume a partnership. To do so would be to override human free will and thus render the soul powerless. This would be against universal law, and nature, on its own, does not live or function outside universal law.

As you told us what your emotional situation was, we observed the energy dynamics as they shifted and moved throughout your system on all PEMS levels. (We see the human system on all PEMS levels because that complete system is functioning in a form state.) We were able to observe the emotional blocks you were struggling with from the perspective of energy. From these observations, we were able to alter the blocks as well as the general movement of energy in a way that assisted and made more efficient that energy's movement. In short, we assisted you in achieving involution/evolution balance in those areas where you had temporarily lost it. As a result, you experienced the shifts, insights, releases and understanding required in the re-establishing of involution/evolution balance throughout your entire system. Remember, we see these blocks from the standpoint of energy—what is moving appropriately and what is not. We see your system as energy relating to form from the perspective of involution/evolution balance. We do not define what results in insights, understanding and resolution. This is the evolutionary input and thrust for which **you** are responsible.

Our process with you is an example both of the partnership we seek with humans and how we can work together in every way to achieve full, inspirited, functioning form. Where the will of the human is present, and where we of nature have been requested to help, we will adjust, shift and facilitate the involution systems in order to support the human's evolution process. For us, it is a relatively simple matter to work with you in this way. In fact, it is solely a matter of receiving a person's request for our assistance.

We suggest that we work together using the following process.

CALIBRATION PROCESS STEPS

1. Open a Healing Coning: Deva of Healing, Pan, a link with the White Brotherhood, your higher self.

NOTE: *We recommend that flower essences be used in this process. We suggest that the person test for essences after opening the coning and prior to stating the problem. This will stabilize the person throughout the process. A dosage need not be tested for, since any essences needed in the beginning of the process will be for short-term stabilization.*

2. Request assistance with a problem that is primarily focused on the emotional or mental levels.

3. State the problem. State it as if you were telling a therapist. Talk about the problem itself and how it is affecting you physically, emotionally, mentally and/or spiritually.

4. Once you have given a full description, allow yourself approximately a half-hour to move through insight, release, understanding and resolution stages.

NOTE: You may not perceive any changes in attitude or understanding during the half-hour. This will be because the process of shifting understanding and changes in attitude sometimes needs to move through more complex levels in order to reach a point where one can perceive the effects. We suggest that if you have sat quietly for a half-hour and no sense of understanding or resolution has come to you, simply move forward in faith that very shortly, within twenty-four hours, you will experience understanding, change and resolution.

5. We suggest that you test for flower essences again just prior to closing the coning and include a dosage/solution test for continued support during the integration process.

6. Close the coning by asking to be disconnected from each member of the coning, one at a time. Test, using kinesiology, to make sure the coning is closed. (If you test negative after asking if it is closed, just refocus on the coning and again request to be disconnected from each member, one at a time. You simply lost your focus the first time. After the second time, you will test positive.)

*ADDITIONAL NOTES: We see some emotional/mental problems as comparatively complex layerings of energy movement. It is quite possible that for the **final** resolution of an emotional/mental issue, one will need to go through this process several times. But we also stress that timing is a key* *factor. If and when a follow-up session is needed, you will sense something related to the original problem that has become an issue. One need not plan ahead for these follow-ups, for you will need time between sessions to integrate the insight, release, understanding and resolution from the previous session.*

The half-hour timing more than covers the time span we need to move the human system through involution/evolution imbalance into involution/evolution balance. Don't forget that in the more complex situations, you will be moving through a series of sessions with us that will resemble the peeling process or two-week process described in the book, Flower Essences. You will move through one layer at a time, experiencing a sense of resolution after each layer, which, once integrated, will signal you to move on to the next layer.

For a twenty-four hour period of time after a calibration, you may feel tired and a little quiet—even feel an ache or pain that has seemingly popped up from nowhere. These are simply reactions to the calibration and should be gone within twenty-four hours. The integration-period flower essences solution will assist and stabilize you greatly through this twenty-four hour period. However, if a reaction should persist, set up another Calibration Process around the same issue and explain all of the various reactions you are having. Nature will do additional adjustments that will either move you through or eliminate the reactions.

The Calibration Process is an additional nature-partnership procedure that is not in and of itself strictly a flower essence process. With or without the essences, this process can work. Flower essences would be most helpful, however, in stabilizing you throughout the Calibration Process itself and afterwards during the time needed for integrating the work accomplished during the process.

COMBINING CALIBRATION WITH MAP

The Calibration Process stands on its own and does not need to be combined with MAP. To do a Calibration Process on its own, simply follow the steps as outlined in the session above. However, for those of us who wish to work with MAP or are already working with it, it is more efficient to combine the two processes. By pointing out the differences in the two processes, I think you will more easily see why they are both complementary and advantageous for us to use.

When we are in a MAP session, we are in a coning that links us to our medical team and stabilizes that link throughout the entire session. Nature is a part of that coning and is essential in maintaining the link and stabilization while the team works with us. The work is done primarily between us and our Brotherhood team.

In a Calibration Process, nature becomes an active team member in addition to its linking and stabilizing role. Nature, through Pan, shifts and adjusts us *physically* into an alignment that enhances and facilitates emotional and mental process. When we think about it, linked with every challenge we face is emotional and mental process.

When I am in a MAP session in which I have combined the Calibration Process, I feel as if my medical team is working with me on one level and Pan is in a closer, physical proximity to me and working *in concert* with the medical team to move me physically through the session. The work done in a MAP session is efficient beyond belief. But what is accomplished in a combination MAP/Calibration session takes efficiency to the point of an art form. The Brotherhood Medical Unit loves it and truly appreciates working with nature in such a direct way. Because of their deference to our timing, they cannot initiate this combination for us. We must take responsibility for expanding MAP sessions to include nature in a direct, working partnership with us and the MAP team. Now, it is rare that I have a MAP session without setting Calibration up in it.

I suggest that you try the Calibration Process on its own for a few times just to get used to how it feels. Then, combine it with the MAP sessions. There will be times when you will know that you do not need a full MAP/Calibration session. You need only the Calibration Process.

Here's how to include the Calibration Process with MAP.

1. Open the MAP session as usual, activating the MAP coning. Test yourself for essences, if they are part of your program.

2. State:

> I'd like also to open to Pan for the Calibration Process. I'd like that connection to occur now.

Wait 5-10 seconds for this connection. Pan, who is already part of the MAP coning, will shift from that coning dynamic and move into a connection with you that is appropriate for the Calibration Process. You may or may not feel this shift. It is unimportant either way. If you use kinesiology, you can verify your connection with Pan for Calibration.

3. Now, explain to both your team and Pan what your difficulty is. You will be working together in a three-level team: you, Pan and the Brotherhood medical team. Continue through the MAP session as you normally would. Allow the session to last the full 40 minutes.

4. When the session is complete, thank everyone and close down the coning. You will disconnect from:
   Overlighting Deva of Healing
   Pan: *from within the Calibration Process link*
   Pan: *from within the coning*
   White Brotherhood: Medical Unit
   Your higher self

5. Test yourself for essences and dosage. Spend a few minutes quietly before going on with your day.

Chapter 6

Easy Reference Steps for MAP and MAP/Calibration

 FIRST SESSION: THE SCANNING SESSION

1. Lie on your back with a blanket close at hand.

2. Open the coning. State:
   I'd like to open a MAP coning. I'd like to connect with:

   > Overlighting Deva of Healing
   > Pan
   > White Brotherhood: Medical Unit
   > My higher self

3. Scanning: You do not need to talk. Remain still for 1 hour. At the end of the hour, request that you be given a symbol or word or sensation to be used as identification for your team.

4. Close the coning. Spend a few minutes quietly.

Wait 24 hours before the second session.

REGULAR SESSIONS

1. Lie down with a blanket and have the flower essences handy.

2. Open a MAP coning:
   Overlighting Deva of Healing
   Pan
   White Brotherhood: Medical Unit (Visualize or say your identification code.)
   Your higher self

3. Test essences.

4. Focus attention on the medical team and describe fully how you are feeling. Tell them everything that comes to mind. Give feedback on any sensations you feel during the session. Session lasts 40 minutes.

5. At the end of 40 minutes, thank your team and close the session by closing the coning. Disconnect from each member of the coning individually.

6. Test yourself for flower essences and check for dosage. Spend a few minutes quietly.

MAP/CALIBRATION COMBINED SESSIONS

1. Lie down with a blanket and have the flower essences handy.

2. Open a MAP coning:
   Overlighting Deva of Healing
   Pan

White Brotherhood: Medical Unit (Visualize/say your identification code.)
Your higher self

3. Test for essences.

4. State:
I'd like to also open to Pan for the Calibration Process. I'd like that connection to occur now.
Wait 5-10 seconds or kinesiology test to verify.

5. Explain to both your team and Pan what your difficulty is. Describe fully how you are feeling. Tell them everything that comes to mind. Give feedback on any sensations you feel during the session. Combined session lasts 40 minutes.

6. Close the session. Thank everyone and close down the coning by disconnecting from:
Overlighting Deva of Healing
Pan: *from within the Calibration Process link*
Pan: *from within the MAP coning*
Your White Brotherhood medical team
Your higher self

7. Test yourself for essences and dosage. Spend a few minutes quietly.

> NOTE: *Do not do these steps without first reading this book. The information contained in the book is vital to your understanding the process steps.*

IMPORTANT

If you wish to share MAP with others, it is *vital* that you make this book available to them and not just the MAP steps. It is important that anyone using MAP has the information contained in the book to use as a foundation. To give them just the steps would place them at a serious disadvantage, lead to possible misinterpretation of the steps and possibly cause them difficulties. MAP is a potent tool and should not be entered lightly nor should it be shared with others in a haphazard manner.

We ask that MAP not be presented in a group context unless the book is made available to the participants at the time of the presentation. Again, it is important that people have access to the full information about MAP and not have to depend on another person's personal interpretation of the program. Please contact us at Perelandra for details on making the book available.

Also, "for best results, use as directed." The MAP process gives optimal results because it was constructed with a balance between the involutionary (i) dynamic of nature (devas and Pan) and the evolutionary (e) dynamic of the White Brotherhood and the person's higher self. That balance assures you optimal safety, efficiency and results. Changing the process in any way alters the i/e balance with which it was designed to be used, and may therefore affect the results.

Finally, use good judgment about consulting trained health care professionals when needed. MAP can be used in conjunction with a doctor's care. Do not feel you must choose one over the other.

Appendices

Appendix A:

Kinesiology

I have mentioned that one of the best and most effective means for communicating with a Brotherhood medical team is kinesiology. Kinesiology is the fancy name for muscle testing. If you want to get medical information from your team, all you have to do is ask simple yes/no questions that will cover the information that you seek. Your team will project a yes or no into your electrical system and you will then be able to discern their answer by kinesiology. For those of you who already use this method for getting information from nature or for testing the flower essences, you already have the tool in place for communicating with your team. Just direct your questions to your team. But make sure they are in the simple yes/no format. And do the kinesiology test.

For those of you who have never heard of such a thing but would like to try it, I am reprinting the section on developing kinesiology testing from the book, *Flower Essences* .

KINESIOLOGY:
THE TOOL FOR TESTING

Kinesiology is simple. Everybody can do it because it links you to your electrical system and your muscles. If you are alive, you have these two things. I know that sounds smart-mouthed of me, but I've learned that sometimes people refuse to believe anything can be so simple. So they create a mental block—only "sensitive types" can do this, or only women can do this. It's just not true. Kinesiology happens to be one of those simple things in life that's waiting around to be learned and used by everyone.

If you've ever been to a chiropractor or wholistic physician, chances are you've experienced kinesiology. The doctor tells you to stick out your arm and resist his pressure. It feels like he's trying to push your arm down after he's told you not to let him do it. Everything is going fine, and then all of a sudden he presses and your arm falls down like a floppy fish. That's kinesiology.

Let me explain: If negative energy (that is, any physical object or energy that does not maintain or enhance health and balance) is introduced into a person's overall energy field, either within his body or in his immediate environment, his muscles, when having physical pressure applied, are unable to hold their strength. In other words, if pressure is applied to an individual's extended arm while his field is affected by negative energy, the arm will not be able to resist the pressure. It will weaken and fall to his side. In the case of the physician or chiropractor, they are testing specific areas of the body. When making contact with a weakened area, the muscles respond by losing their strength. If pressure is applied while connecting with a positive or balanced area, the person will easily be able to resist and the arm will hold its position.

To expand further, when negative energy is placed within a person's field, his electrical system (that electrical grid that is contained within and around his body) will immediately respond by "short-circuiting." This makes it difficult for the muscles to maintain their strength and hold the position when pressure is added. When positive energy is within the field, the electrical system holds and the muscles maintain their strength when pressure is applied.

This electrical/muscular relationship is a natural part of the human system. It is not mystical or magical. Kinesiology is the established method for reading their balance at any given moment.

If you have ever experienced muscle testing, you most likely participated in the above-described, two-man operation. You provided the extended arm and the other person provided the pressure. Although efficient, this can sometimes be cumbersome when you want to test something on your own. Arm pumpers have the nasty habit of disappearing right when you need them most. So you'll be learning to self-test—no arm pumpers needed.

KINESIOLOGY SELF-TESTING STEPS

1. THE CIRCUIT FINGERS: **If you are right-handed:** Place your left hand palm up. Connect the tip of your 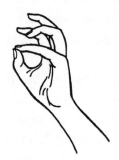 left thumb with the tip of the left little finger (*not your index finger*). If **you are left-handed:** Place your right hand palm up. Connect the tip of your right thumb with the tip of your right little finger. By connecting your thumb and little finger, you have just closed an electrical circuit in your hand, and it is this circuit you will use for testing.

Before going on, look at the position you have just formed with your hand. If your thumb is touching the tip of your index or first finger, laugh at yourself for not being able to follow directions and change the position to touch the tip of the thumb with the tip of the little or fourth finger. Most likely this will not feel at all comfortable to you. If you are feeling a weird sense of awkwardness, you've got the first step of the test position! In time, the hand and fingers will adjust to being put in this position and it will feel fine.

2. THE TEST FINGERS: To test the circuit (the means by which you will apply pressure to yourself), place the thumb and index finger of your other hand inside the circle you have created by connect-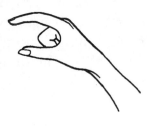

ing your thumb and little finger. The thumb/index finger should be right under the thumb/little finger, touching them. Don't try to make a circle with your test fingers. They're just placed inside the circuit fingers which do form a circle. It will look as if the circuit fingers are resting on the test fingers.

3. POSITIVE RESPONSE: Keeping this position, ask yourself a yes/no question in which you already know the answer to be yes. ("Is my name _____?") Once you've asked the question, press your circuit fingers together, keeping the tip-to-tip position. *Using the same amount of pressure,* try to pull apart the cir- 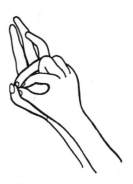 cuit fingers with your test fingers. Press the lower thumb against the upper thumb, the lower index finger against the upper little finger.

Another way to say all this is that the circuit position described in Step 1 corresponds to the position you take when you stick your arm out for the physician. The testing position in Step 2 is in place of the physician or other convenient arm pumper. After you ask the yes/no question and you press your circuit fingers tip-to-tip, that's equal to the doctor saying, "Resist my pressure." Your circuit fingers now correspond to your outstretched, stiffened arm. Trying to pull apart those fingers with your testing fingers is equal to the doctor pressing down on your arm.

83

If the answer to the question is positive (if your name is what you think it is!), you will not be able to easily pull apart the circuit fingers. The electrical circuit will hold, your muscles will maintain their strength, and your circuit fingers will not separate. You will feel the strength in that circuit. *Important: Be sure the amount of pressure holding the circuit fingers together is equal to the amount your testing fingers press against them. Also, don't use a pumping action in your testing fingers when trying to pry your circuit fingers apart. Use an equal, steady and continuous pressure.*

Play with this a bit. Ask a few more yes/no questions that have positive answers. Now, I know it's going to seem that if you already know the answer to be yes, you are probably "throwing" the test. That's reasonable, but for the time being, until you get a feeling for what the positive response feels like in your fingers, you're going to need to deliberately ask yourself questions with positive answers.

While asking questions, if you are having trouble sensing the strength of the circuit, apply a little more pressure. Or consider that you may be applying too much pressure and pull back some. You don't have to break or strain your fingers for this; just use enough pressure to make them feel alive, connected and alert.

4. NEGATIVE RESPONSE: Once you have a clear sense of the positive response, ask yourself a question that has a negative answer. Again press your circuit fingers together and, *using equal pressure*, press against the circuit fingers with the test fingers. This time the electrical

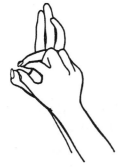

circuit will break and the circuit fingers will weaken and separate. Because the electrical circuit is broken, the muscles in the circuit fingers don't have the power to hold the fingers together. In a positive state, the electrical circuit holds and the muscles have the power to keep the two fingers together.

Play with negative questions a bit, and then return to positive questions. Get a good feeling for the strength between your circuit fingers when the electricity is in a positive state and the weakness when the electricity is in a negative state. You can even ask yourself (your own system) for a positive response and then, after testing, ask for a negative response. ("Give me a positive response." Test. "Give me a negative response." Test.) You will feel the positive strength and the negative weakness. In the beginning, you may feel only a slight difference between the two. With practice, that difference will become more pronounced. For now, it's just a matter of trusting what you've learned—and practice.

Don't forget the overall concept behind kinesiology. What enhances our body, mind and soul makes us strong. Together, our body, mind and soul create a wholistic environment which, when balanced, is strong and solid. If something enters that environment and negates or challenges the balance, the entire environment is weakened. That strength or weakness registers in the electrical system, and it can be discerned through the muscle testing technique—kinesiology.

KINESIOLOGY TIPS

If you are having trouble feeling the electrical circuit on the circuit fingers, try switching hands—the circuit fingers become the testing fingers and vice versa. Most people who are right-handed have this particular electrical circuitry in their left hand. Left-handers generally have the circuitry in their right hand. But sometimes a right-hander has the circuitry in the right hand and a left-hander has it in the left hand. You may be one of those people.

If you have an injury such as a muscle sprain in either hand or arm, don't try to learn kinesiology until you have healed. Kinesiology is muscle testing, and a muscle injury will interfere with the testing—and the testing will interfere with the healing of the muscle injury.

Also, when first learning kinesiology, do yourself a favor and set aside some quiet time to go through the instructions and play with the testing. Trying to learn this while riding the New York subway during evening rush hour isn't going to give you the break you need. But once you have learned it, you'll be able to test all kinds of things while riding the subway.

Sometimes I meet people who are trying to learn kinesiology and aren't having much luck. They've gotten frustrated, decided this isn't for them, and have gone on to try to learn another means of testing. Well, I'll listen to them explain what they did, and before they know it, I've verbally tricked them with a couple of suggestions about their testing, which they try, and they begin feeling kinesiology for the first time—a strong 'yes' and a clear 'no.' The problem wasn't kinesiology. Everyone, as I have said, has an electrical system. The problem was that they wanted to learn it so much that they became overly anxious and tense—they blocked.

So, since you won't have me around to trick you, I suggest that if you suspect you're blocking, go on to something else. Then trick yourself. When you care the least about whether or not you learn kinesiology, start playing with it again. Approach it as if it were a game. *Then* you'll feel the strength and weakness in the fingers.

Now, suppose the testing has been working fine, and then suddenly you can't get a clear result (what I call a "definite maybe") or get no result at all. Check:

1. Sloppy testing. You try to press apart the fingers before applying pressure between the circuit fingers. This happens especially when we've been testing for awhile and become over-confident or do the testing very quickly. I think it happens to all of us from time to time and serves to remind us to keep our attention on the matter at hand. (Excuse the lousy pun.)

2. External distractions. Trying to test in a noisy or active area can cause you to lose concentration. The testing will feel unsure or contradict itself if you double-check the results. Often, simply moving to a quiet, calm spot

and concentrating on what you are doing will be just what's needed for successful testing.

3. Focus/concentration. Even in a quiet spot, one's mind may wander and the testing will feel fuzzy, weak or contradictory. It's important to concentrate throughout the process. Check how you are feeling. If you're tired, I suggest you not try to test until you've rested a bit. And if you have to go to the bathroom, do it. That little situation is a sure concentration-destroyer.

4. The question isn't clear. A key to kinesiology is asking a *simple* yes/no question, not two questions in one, each having a possible yes/no answer. When testing for flower essences, make sure you ask one question at a time.

5. You must want to accept the results of the test. If you enter a kinesiology test not wanting to "hear" the answer, for whatever reason, you can override the test with your emotions and your will. This is true for conventional situations as well. If you really don't want something to work for you, it won't work. That's our personal power dictating the outcome.

Also, if you are trying to do testing during a situation that is especially emotional for you, that deeply stirs your emotions, or if you are trying to ask a question in which you have a strong, personal investment in the answer—such as, "Should I buy this beautiful $250,000 house?"—I suggest that you not test until you are calmer or get some emotional distance from the situation. During such times, you're walking a very fine line between a clear test and a test that your desires are over-riding. Kinesiology as a tool isn't the issue here. It's the condition or intent of the tester. In fact, some questions just shouldn't be asked, but *which questions* are relative to who's doing the asking. We each need to develop discernment around which questions are appropriate for us to ask.

If you are in an emergency situation, for example, and have no choice but to test someone close who might need flower essences, be aware of your emotional vulnerability. When I am involved with testing during emotionally stressful times, I stop for a moment, collect my thoughts and make a commitment to concentrate on the testing only. If I need to test an emotionally charged question or a question about something I have a personal investment in, I stop a moment, commit myself to the test and open myself to receiving *the* answer and not the answer I might desire.

A NOTE ON CLARITY

If you're having difficulty wording a simple yes/no question, consider this an important issue to be faced and something worth spending time to rectify. You have not simply stumbled upon a glitch in your quest to use kinesiology. You've also stumbled upon a glitch in the communication between your higher self and your conscious self. If you can't even clearly phrase the question, you can't expect an answer. I have met people who cannot articulate a question. In a workshop they will attempt to ask me something and I can't figure out what they are asking—nor can anyone else in the workshop. Usually it turns out that they are frustrated because they can't get any clarity in their own life and are trying to ask me what to do about it.

For those of you who find yourselves in this boat, you have a terrific opportunity to turn that around and develop internal order by learning how to articulate a simple yes/no question. If you do this, you not only develop the tool of kinesiology, you also develop clarity for communicating with yourself. I fully understand that it will take focus on your part, and in comparison to someone who finds articulating a simple question easy, to you it will seem herculean. But if you wish to function consciously on your many levels, you must have internal clarity and order.

I recommend that you initially devote your attention to learning to ask simple questions and not worry about receiving answers. When you need to ask someone a question, take time to consider what you really want to ask and how it can be most clearly and efficiently worded. It helps to write down the question. In this way, you can visually see your words. If they don't convey what you mentally want to express, play with the wording. Keep doing this until you feel those words accurately and concisely communicate what you wish to ask. Then go to that person and ask the question. Notice the difference in quality of how the person answers you. Your clarity will inspire similar clarity in the response.

I urge you to continue this process for a fair period of time—even dedicating yourself to the process for awhile. Quite often, that frustrating inner confusion exists because we've not had an acceptable framework for the development of mental ordering. Learning to ask questions gives the mind something tangible to work with and, in the process, you learn mind-word-and-mouth coordination. You'll find that as you develop the ability to clearly articulate a question, your inner fog will begin to lift, which in turn will automatically begin to lift your outer fog.

FINAL COMMENTS ON KINESIOLOGY

Kinesiology is like any tool. The more you practice, the better you are at using it. You need a sense of confidence about using this tool, especially when you get some very strange answers to what you thought were pretty straight questions. It helps you get over the initial "this-is-weird-and-the-damned-testing-isn't-working" stage if you have some confidence in your ability to feel clear positive and negative responses. The only way I know over this hump is to practice testing. You will develop clarity in your testing and you'll learn your personal pitfalls.

In teaching kinesiology, I have found that something interesting happens to some people when they are learning it. Every block, doubt, question and personal challenge they have, when faced head-on with something perceived as unconventional, comes right to the surface. It's as if the physical tool of kinesiology itself serves to bring to the surface all those hurdles. So they learn kinesiology right away and are using it well. Then, all of a sudden it's not working for them. When they tell me about it, I realize that the thing they do differently now that they didn't do at first is double-checking their answers—and rechecking, and rechecking, and doing it again, and again . . . Each time the answers vary or the fingers get mushy and they get definite maybe's.

Well, again the issue isn't the kinesiology. The issue is really why they are suddenly doing all this rechecking business. What have surfaced for them are questions around trust in their own ability, belief that such unconventional things really do happen and are happening to them, and a sudden lack of self-confidence.

The only way I know to get over this hurdle is to defy it—keep testing. The other alternative is to succumb and stop developing with kinesiology. But, that doesn't really accomplish anything. So in cases like this, I suggest the person keep testing, *stop* double-checking and take the plunge to go with his first test result. Eventually, what is done based on the first test result will verify the accuracy of the test. From this, your confidence builds. I firmly believe that only clear personal evidence can get us through these kinds of hurdles and blocks—and that means just continuing to go on.

So, what can we practice test on? Everything. You could easily drive yourself nuts. What colors you should wear. What colors you should wear for a special event.

What would be healthiest for you to eat for breakfast, lunch and dinner. You take ten separate vitamin and mineral supplements as a matter of course on a daily basis. Try testing them individually. ("Do I need vitamin E? B6? Iron?") to see if you need all ten every day. Or if there are some you don't need to take at all. You are sitting at a restaurant and they don't have Tofu Supreme on the menu. Is there anything on that menu that is healthy for you to eat? ("Should I eat fish?" [yes/no] "Should I eat beef?" [yes/no] "Chicken?" [yes/no] "Häagen-Dazs fudge ripple ice cream?!") And one thing you can frequently test yourself for is whether or not you need flower essences.

The point is to test everything you possibly can that doesn't place you in a life-threatening situation, follow through on your answers and then look at the results. As I have worked through the years to refine my ability to use kinesiology, I have, on many occasions, purposely followed through on answers that made no sense at all to me, just to see if the testing was accurate. Doing this and looking at the results with a critical eye is the only way I know to learn about ourselves as kinesiology testers and to discover the nuances and uses of kinesiology itself.

One last piece of information: Give yourself about a year to develop confidence with kinesiology. Now, you'll be able to use it right away. This just takes sticking with your initial efforts until you get those first feelings of positive strength and negative weakness in the circuit fingers. But I have found from my own experience and from watching others that it takes about a year of experimentation to fully learn the art of asking accurate yes/no questions, and to overcome the hurdles. As one woman said, "You stick with this stuff a year, and boy, what a great thing you end up with!"

Appendix B

FLOWER ESSENCES

For those of you who would like to know more about flower essences, I am reprinting the section on flower essences from the Perelandra Catalog. As part of the co-creative garden work here at Perelandra, we produce two sets of flower essences: Perelandra Rose Essences and Perelandra Garden Essences. There are a number of flower essences available in the United States, Great Britain and Australia and it is unimportant to me and to MAP which essences you use. So I offer you the Perelandra information in the spirit of giving you general information about flower essences and specific information about the Perelandra essences. At the end of Appendix B is a list of other flower essences suppliers who will be happy to send you their catalogs on request.

From the Perelandra Catalog:

The human body has within and surrounding it an electrical network. When we experience health, this electrical network is balanced and fully connected. When something in our life or environment threatens that balance, the electrical system responds by either short-circuiting or overloading. That imbalance in the electrical system immediately impacts the central nervous system. The body then goes into high gear in an effort to correct the imbalance. If our body does not succeed, we physically manifest the imbalance. We get a cold or a headache or our allergy pops up again or another migraine belts us. Or we get back pain or our neck goes out again. Or we become seriously ill.

Flower essences work directly with both the electrical and the central nervous systems. By taking the correct essences, we immediately balance the electrical system, stabilize the nervous system and stop the domino effect that leads to illness.

If we don't take the essences and wind up getting sick, we can still take the essence(s) which will then stabilize and balance the electrical and nervous systems while the body gets on with the business of fighting off the problem. By assisting this process, flower essences drastically reduce our recovery time. In short, by using the essences, we are not asking our body to pull double duty— work to heal us systemically *and* rebalance our electrical and central nervous systems.

A different perspective about the essences, excerpted from a session given by the Deva of Flower Essences in the book, *Flower Essences,* might be helpful:

> *. . . You are getting the idea that all is changing. How one perceives his health is also changing. As with everything around him, the key to this change is balance. One's health will be intimately linked with one's understanding and response to balance.*

. . . *They* [flower essences] *support and help secure balance on all levels—physical, emotional, mental and spiritual. Physically, they balance the body by reconnecting and adjusting the electrical system. Emotionally and mentally, they help the person identify, alter and sometimes remove emotional and mental patterns that challenge his overall balance. And spiritually, they assist the person's connection to and understanding of the many levels of himself so that he can operate in life from a broader perspective.*

Flower essences provide a health system that is aligned to both the surrounding universal dynamics of transition, and the individual's expansion and response to the times by having incorporated within the system itself the key to it all— balance.

The Perelandra flower essences have been a natural development in the work that has gone on between nature and myself. They are produced from the flowers, vegetables and herbs grown in the Perelandra garden. The essences are carefully prepared and stabilized pattern-infused water tinctures that are then preserved in brandy. The tinctures go through a final stabilization inside the genesa crystal sitting in the center of the garden. They are bottled in a concentrate form in pharmaceutical dropper bottles that make it easy and convenient for you to place one drop of a needed essence directly on your tongue or several drops of the essence in a glass of water to be sipped throughout the day.

I feel that through these flower essences we at Perelandra are able to share the extraordinary vitality and power that has resulted from the co-creative work with nature in the Perelandra garden. In using the essences, we establish another partnership with nature—this one focused on our health, balance and well-being.

If you are intrigued, interested or curious about flower essences and wish to investigate them further, I offer some suggestions on how you might proceed without feeling overwhelmed.

✳ Read *Flower Essences: Reordering Our Understanding and Approach to Illness and Health.* It will give you a crystal-clear idea about what flower essences are, the testing techniques and processes used, how to choose the essences you need and suggestions on how to successfully integrate them into your life. The Perelandra essences are fully discussed, but the book is applicable to all flower essences and presents step-by-step processes that can be used for any essences on the market. (If you already have a set of essences and wish to use them with greater effectiveness and precision, you might consider getting the book, *Flower Essences.*)

✳ For those who would like to try essences and experience how they work: Read through the Perelandra essence definitions that are listed in this appendix. Then think about some physical, emotional, mental or spiritual problem you would like to address. Think of it clearly or even write it out. Then say to yourself, "What essence(s) do I need to help me with this problem now?" Read through the definitions again and note which one(s) *intuitively* pop out to you. (If you know kinesiology, you can simply test the list of essences, choosing the ones which test positive for you.) Order the essences that stand out when you read the definitions. (Try to keep your rational mind out of the process!) You'll get a Guide with the bottles which will explain how to use them and teach you how to find out how often to take them. Usually one drop, once or twice daily for several days will do the trick. Then see how you feel. Also, get the book *Flower Essences* so that you can see more clearly when and how they are to be used.

✻ For those, like myself, who are immediately struck between the eyes by these things called "flower essences" and know they belong in your life: I strongly suggest that you purchase the complete set of Perelandra essences. That is, both the Rose Essences set and the Garden Essences set. Now, to be honest with you, I've been reluctant to suggest this to people. I'm sensitive to the fact that we're talking about money here and, as the producer/developer of the Perelandra essences, there is an obvious conflict of interest in my suggestion. But this year I feel urged to come out of the closet with this suggestion for three reasons:

1. These two sets often work in *combination* with one another. The Rose Essences address and support the various steps we move through as we face overall

change and transition. The Garden Essences address specific issues on the physical, emotional, mental and spiritual levels that either trigger transition or arise because of transition. In my work as an essence practitioner, I have found that often a person needs support for both the transition process itself and the specific issues coming up due to the process.

2. The complete set of Perelandra essences covers a full range of transition issues and specific issues. What is needed this week will often be different from what is needed next week or next month or next year. The essences are used one or two drops at a time and have an indefinite shelf life. In short, you'll be keeping and using the set for many years. It's fair to assume that you or someone close to you will be needing each of the essences at some point. It's more convenient to have them on hand when needed rather than have to order those specific bottles and wait for them to arrive in the mail before using them.

3. I've noticed over the past years that a fair number of people initially ordering single bottles or partial sets end up ordering the complete set. After using them, they came to the conclusion that to use the essences with the greatest of agility and accuracy, one needs to have on hand the full range provided by the complete set of Perelandra essences.

I also suggest that when ordering the complete set of Perelandra essences, you include *Flower Essences* along with your order. I know I am suggesting this book a lot.

But I feel strongly that it will help you to organize and integrate the essences into your life in a precise and extremely effective manner.

As I've mentioned, there are two different sets of Perelandra flower essences: the Perelandra Rose Essences and the Perelandra Garden Essences. With each purchase, individual bottles or sets, you also get the Guide which gives the step-by-step basic processes for accurately testing yourself for the essences you need and discerning the correct dosage—how many drops of the essences are needed for how many days. Also included in the Guide are the long definitions for each of the essences. Reading them will give you a clearer idea of what the essences address.

THE PERELANDRA ROSE ESSENCES

The Perelandra Rose Essences are a set of eight flower essences. Made from roses in the Perelandra garden, these eight essences function with one another to support and balance an individual's physical body and soul as he proceeds forward. As we experience expansion or move forward in process, there are mechanisms within us which are set in motion to facilitate our periods of growth. The Perelandra Rose Essences help to stabilize and balance us and our expansion mechanisms.

The following are short definitions of the Perelandra Rose Essences. The name of each essence is the same as the rose from which it is made.

GRUSS AN AACHEN: Stability. Balances and stabilizes the body/soul unit on all PEMS levels (physical, emotional, mental, spiritual) as it moves forward in its evolutionary process.

PEACE: Courage. Opens the individual to the inner dynamic of courage that is aligned to universal courage.

ECLIPSE: Acceptance and insight. Enhances the individual's appreciation of his own inner knowing. Supports the mechanism which allows the body to receive the soul's input and insight.

ORANGE RUFFLES: Receptivity. Stabilizes the individual during the expansion of his sensory system.

AMBASSADOR: Pattern. Aids the individual in seeing the relationship of the part to the whole, in perceiving his pattern and purpose.

NYMPHENBURG: Strength. Supports and holds the strength created by the balance of the body/soul fusion, and facilitates the individual's ability to regain that balance.

WHITE LIGHTNIN': Synchronized movement. Stabilizes the inner timing of all PEMS levels moving in concert, and enhances the body/soul fusion.

ROYAL HIGHNESS: Final stabilization. The mop-up essence which helps to insulate, protect and stabilize the individual and to stabilize the shift during its final stages while vulnerable.

THE PERELANDRA GARDEN ESSENCES

This set of eighteen essences is made from the flower petals of vegetables, herbs and flowers grown in the Perelandra garden. Their balancing and restorative patterns address physical, emotional, mental and spiritual issues that we face in today's world.

BROCCOLI: For the power balance which must be maintained when one perceives himself to be under seige from outside. Stabilizes the body/soul unit so the person won't close down, detach and scatter.

CAULIFLOWER: Stabilizes and balances the child during the birth process.

CELERY: Restores balance of the immune system during times when it is being overworked or stressed, and during long-term viral or bacterial infections.

CHIVES: Re-establishes the power one has when the internal male/female dynamics are balanced and the person is functioning in a state of awareness within this balance.

COMFREY: Repairs higher vibrational soul damage that occurred in the present or a past lifetime.

CORN: Stabilization during universal/spiritual expansion. Assists transition of experience into useful, pertinent understanding and action.

CUCUMBER: Rebalancing during depression. Vital re-attachment to life.

DILL: Assists individual in reclaiming power balance one has released to others. Victimization.

NASTURTIUM: Restores vital physical life energy during times of intense mental-level focus.

OKRA: Returns ability to see the positive in one's life and environment.

SALVIA: Restores emotional stability during times of extreme stress.

SNAP PEA: Rebalances child or adult after a nightmare. Assists in ability to translate daily experience into positive, understandable process.

SUMMER SQUASH: Restores courage to the person who experiences fear and resistance when faced with daily routine. Shyness. Phobia.

SWEET BELL PEPPER: Inner peace, clarity and calm when faced with today's stressful times. Stabilizes body/soul balance during times of stress.

TOMATO: Cleansing. Assists the body in shattering and throwing off that which is causing infection or disease.

YELLOW YARROW: Emotional protection during vulnerable times. Its support softens resistance and assists the integration process.

ZINNIA: Reconnects one to the child within. Restores playfulness, laughter, joy and a sense of healthy priorities.

ZUCCHINI: Helps restore physical strength during con-
valescence.

_____

OTHER FLOWER ESSENCES SOURCES

Flower Essence Services
P.O. Box 586
Nevada City, CA   95959
Tele: 916/273-6363

Alaskan Flower Essence Project
P.O. Box 1369
Homer, AK   99603
Tele: 907/235-2188

PERELANDRA ESSENCES
PURCHASING INFORMATION

BASIC SET: Perelandra Rose & Garden Essences. Both full sets purchased together. Complete sets available in 1-dram (1/8 oz.) and half-ounce bottles.

BASIC SET WITH BOOK: Both sets of Perelandra essences plus the book, *Flower Essences: Reordering Our Understanding and Approach to Illness and Health.* Essences available in 1-dram and half-ounce bottles.

PERELANDRA ROSE ESSENCES SET: Includes eight boxed, *half-ounce dropper bottles*, the Guide and the short-definitions card which may be taped to the inside of the box lid for easy reference.

PERELANDRA GARDEN ESSENCES SET: Two boxes containing a total of eighteen *half-ounce dropper bottles*, the Guide and two short-definitions cards.

PERELANDRA GARDEN ESSENCES SET OF NINE: Nine *half-ounce bottles* of Perelandra Garden Essences *of your choice.* Each set includes a box, the Guide and the short-definitions cards for the inner box lid. Check the list on the order form for choice of essences. (Choice does not include the Perelandra Rose Essences.)

INDIVIDUAL ESSENCES: *Half-ounce dropper bottles* numbering less than nine, plus the Guide.

For prices, new products and ordering information, see p. 128 and the order form at the end of the book.

106

Appendix C

A Bit about Perelandra and My Research with Nature

Perelandra is both home for Clarence and me and a nature research center. It now consists of thirty-three acres of mostly woods in the foothills of the Blue Ridge Mountains in Virginia. The nature research and development has been going on since 1976, when I dedicated myself to learning about nature in new ways from nature itself. I began working with nature intelligences in a coordinated, co-creative and educational effort which has resulted in understanding and demonstrating a new approach to agriculture and ecological balance. Besides publishing materials about the research, we hold an annual workshop series and open house at Perelandra. *Except for these scheduled days, Perelandra is closed to the public in order to have the time and space needed for the continuing research work.*

The primary focus of my work has been the one-hundred-foot-diameter circular garden where I get from nature the information and direction I need to create an all-inclusive garden environment based on the principles of energy in balance. For example, we do not attempt to repel insects. Instead, we focus on creating a balanced environment that calls to it and fully supports a complete and appropriate population of insects. In turn, the insects relate to the garden's plant life in a light and nondestructive manner.

From this kind of work has developed a new method of gardening which I call "co-creative gardening." Briefly, this is a method of gardening in partnership with the nature intelligences that emphasizes balance and teamwork. The balance is a result of concentrating on the laws of the life energy behind form. The teamwork is established between the individual and the intelligent levels inherent in nature. Both of these point out the differences between co-creative gardening and agriculture and traditional organic gardening and agricultural methods. (Information about this work is described in three books: *Behaving As If the God In All Life Mattered*, *Perelandra Garden Workbook: A Complete Guide to Gardening with Nature Intelligences*, and *Perelandra Garden Workbook II: Co-Creative Energy Processes for Gardening, Agriculture and Life*.)

The foundation of the work going on at Perelandra, as I have indicated, comes from nature intelligences, a collective term I use for devas and nature spirits. My work with flower essences and a number of physical health and balancing processes have also been directed from these levels. Therefore, it would be helpful if I gave you an idea of who and what these intelligences are.

"Deva" is a sanskrit word used to describe the intelligent level of consciousness within nature that functions in an architectural mode within all that is form and also serves as the organizer of all that is a part of each form. This means that if I should want to understand or change something in the botanical makeup of a plant species, I would consult with the deva of that species for clarification regarding my specific questions and for advice as to whether my change is viable and ecologically sound. The deva of each type of plant holds the architectural blueprints of that plant and has the power to change the blueprints at any time.

"Nature spirit" refers to the intelligent level of consciousness within nature that works in partnership with the devic level and is responsible for the fusing and maintaining of energy to appropriate five-senses form. Nature spirits tend to the shifting of an energy reality that has been formulated on the devic level and assist the translation of that reality from a dynamic of energy to five-senses form. They also function in a custodial capacity with all that is form on the planet.

To help you understand the work at Perelandra and why nature plays an important and direct role in our health and well-being generally, and MAP and the Calibration Process specifically, I include, in Appendix D, a series of definitions that were given to me by nature. I feel that once you read them you'll sense nature's important role in human health more clearly.

Appendix D

Co-Creative Definitions by Nature and Friends

Let us give you the basic understanding of these terms. We feel that these definitions, kept short and simple, will be more helpful than lengthy, detailed ones. Consider these definitions to be starting points.

❋ **FORM:** *We consider reality to be in the form state when there is organization, order and life vitality combined with a state of consciousness. For the purpose of understanding form in a constructive and workable manner, let us say that we consider consciousness to be soul-initiated and, therefore, quite capable of function beyond what we would term "form." There are dimensions of reality in which the interaction of life reality is maintained on the level of consciousness only. There is no surrounding organization, order or life vitality as we know it. There is only consciousness.*

We do not consider form to be only that which is perceptible to the five senses. In fact, we see form from this perspective to be most limited, both in its life reality and in its ability to function. We see form from the perspective of the five senses to be useful only for the most basic and fundamental level of identification. From this perspective, there is very little

111

relationship to the full understanding and knowledge of how a unit or form system functions.

*All energy contains order, organization and life vitality; therefore, **all energy is form**. If one were to use the term "form" to identify that which can be perceived by the basic senses and the word "energy" to refer to that aspect of an animal, human, plant or object's reality that cannot be readily perceived by the basic senses, then one would be accurate in the use of these two words. However, if one were to use the word "form" to refer to that which can be perceived by the basic five senses and assume form to be a complete unit of reality unto itself, and use the word "energy" to refer to a level beyond form, one would then be using these two words inaccurately.*

On the planet Earth, the personality, character, emotional makeup, intellectual capacity, strong points and gifts of a human are all form. They are that which gives order, organization and life vitality to consciousness.

Order and organization are the physical structures that create a framework for form. In short, they define the walls. But we have included the dynamic of life vitality when we refer to form because one of the elements of form is action, and it is the life vitality that initiates and creates action.

✳ **Nature:** *In the larger universe and beyond, on its many levels and dimensions, there are a number of groups of consciousnesses which, although equal in importance, are quite different in expression and function. Do not misunderstand us by thinking that we are saying that all reality is human soul-oriented but that there are some aspects of this* *reality that function and express differently. We are not saying this. We are saying that there are different groups of consciousnesses that are equal in importance but express and function very differently. Together, they comprise the full expression of the larger, total life picture. No one piece, no one expression, can be missing or the larger life picture on all its levels and dimensions will cease to exist. One such consciousness has been universally termed "nature." Because of what we are saying about the larger picture not existing without all of its parts, you may assume that nature as both a reality and a consciousness exists on all dimensions and all levels. It cannot be excluded.*

Each group of consciousnesses has what can be termed as an area of expertise. As we said, all groups are equal in importance but express and function differently from one another. These different expressions and functions are vital to the overall balance of reality. A truly symbiotic relationship exists among the groups and is based on balance—universal balance. You are absolutely correct to characterize the human soul-oriented dynamic as evolution in scope and function. And you are correct in identifying the nature dynamic as being involution in scope and function. Nature is a massive, intelligent consciousness group that expresses and functions within the many areas of involution, that is, moving soul-oriented consciousness into any dimension or level of form.

*Nature **is** the conscious reality that supplies order, organization and life vitality for this shift. Nature is the consciousness that is, for your working understanding, intimately linked with form. Nature is the consciousness that comprises all form on all levels and dimensions. It is form's order,* *organization and life vitality. Nature is first and foremost a consciousness of equal importance with all other consciousnesses in the largest scheme of reality. It expresses and functions uniquely in that it comprises all form on all levels and dimensions and is responsible for and creates all of form's order, organization and life vitality.*

✳ **Devas and Nature Spirits:** *"Devas" and "nature spirits" are names used to identify two different expressions and functions within the nature consciousness. They are the two groups within the larger nature consciousness that interface with the human soul while in form. There are other groups, and they are differentiated from one another primarily by specific expression and function.*

To expand from our definition of form, it is the devic expression that fuses with consciousness to create order, organization and life vitality. The devic expression as the architect designs the complex order, organization and life vitality that will be needed by the soul consciousness while functioning within the scope or band of form. If the consciousness chooses to shift from one point of form to another point, thereby changing form function, it is the devic expression of nature that alters the organization, order and life vitality accordingly. The devic expression designs and is the creation of the order, organization and life vitality of form.

The nature spirit expression infuses the devic order, organization and life vitality and adds to this the dynamic of function and working balance. To order, organization and life vitality it brings movement and the bond that maintains the alignment of the devic form unit to the universal principles of balance while the consciousness is in form.

*To say that nature is the expert in areas of form and form principles barely scratches the surface of the true nature (pardon the pun) of nature's role in form. It is the expert of form and it is form itself. A soul-oriented consciousness cannot exist on any level or dimension of form in any way without an **equal**, intimate, symbiotic relationship with the nature consciousness.*

✳ **CONSCIOUSNESS:** *The concept of consciousness has been vastly misunderstood. To put it simply, consciousness is the working state of the soul. In human expression, as one sees it demonstrated on the planet Earth, the personality, character, emotional makeup, intellectual capacity, strong points and gifts of a human are all form. They are that which gives order, organization and life vitality to consciousness.*

We say "working state of the soul" because there are levels of soul existence that are different than the working state and can best be described as a simple and complete state of being. The closest that souls on Earth come to this notion is the state of unconsciousness. But this is to give you a glimpse of what we mean by "state of being." We urge you not to assume that what you know as unconsciousness is equal to the soul state of being.

Humans tend to think of the soul as being something that exists far away from them because they are in form. This is an illusion. The core of any life is the soul. It cannot exist apart from itself. Like the heart in the human body, it is an essential part of the life unit. A human in form is, by definition, a soul fused with nature. Personality and character are a part of the nature/form package that allows the soul to function and to express itself in form. They are not the soul; they are the order and organization of that soul.

Consciousness physically fuses into the body system first through the electrical system and then through the central nervous system and the brain. This is another aspect of nature supplying order, organization and life vitality. Consciousness itself cannot be measured or monitored as a reality. But what can be measured and monitored is the order, organization and life vitality of consciousness. Consciousness is the working state of the soul and is not form. It is nature, not consciousness, that supplies form.

We wish to add a thought here so that there will be no confusion about the relationship between nature and the soul. The devic level of nature does not, with its own power, superimpose its interpretation of form onto a soul. We have said that nature and soul are intimately and symbiotically related. This implies a give and take. No one consciousness group operates in isolation of the whole or of all other parts of the whole. When a soul chooses to move within the vast band of form, it communicates its intent and purpose to nature. It is from this that nature, on the devic level, derives the specifics that will be needed for the soul to function in form. It is a perfect marriage of purpose with the order, organization and life vitality that is needed for the fulfillment of that purpose. Nature, therefore, does not define purpose and impose it on a soul. It orders, organizes and gives life vitality to purpose for expression of form.

✳ **SOUL:** *We perceive that most likely the question of soul will arise with anyone reading these definitions. This will be most difficult to define since the soul is, at its point of central essence, beyond form. Consequently, it is beyond words. However, it is not beyond any specific life form. As we have said, an individual is not separate or distant from his or her soul. Souls, as individuated life forces, were created in form at the moment you call the "Big Bang." Beyond form, souls are also beyond the notion of creation. So we refer to the moment of the Big Bang regarding the soul, since this gives you a description of soul that will be most meaningful to you.*

The Big Bang was the nature-designed order, organization and life force used to differentiate soul into sparks of individuated light energy. The power of the Big Bang was created by intent. And that intent originated from the massive collective soul reality beyond form.

It is reasonable to look at the Big Bang as the soul's gateway to the immense band of form. To perceive the soul and how it functions exclusively from the perspective of human form on Earth is akin to seeing that planet from the perspective of one grain of sand. The soul's options of function and expression in form are endless. What we see occurring more frequently now on Earth is the shift from the individual soul unknowingly functioning in an array of options, all chosen only because they are compatible to the immediate purpose of the soul, to the individual beginning to function with discrimination and intent in more expanded ways. Using the words in their more limited, parochial definitions, we can say that we see the beginning of a shift from soul function in which an individuated personality remains unaware of many

117

of its options to soul function in which the personality begins to take on conscious awareness of all its options.

✴ **Energy:** *For those experiencing life on Earth, energy is form that is perceived by an individual beyond the scope of the basic five senses. All energy contains order, organization and life vitality; therefore, **all energy is form**. The makeup and design of the specific order, organization and life vitality within that which can be perceived by the basic five senses is identical to and therefore harmonious with its broader reality, which cannot be perceived by the basic five senses. If one is to use the term "form" to identify that which can be perceived by the basic senses and the word "energy" to refer to that aspect of an animal, human, plant or object's reality that cannot be readily perceived by the basic senses, then one would be accurate in the use of these two words. However, if one is to use the word "form" to refer to that which can be perceived by the basic five senses and assume form to be a complete unit of reality unto itself, and use the word "energy" to refer to a level beyond form, one would then be using these two words inaccurately. From our perspective, form and energy create one unit of reality and are differentiated from one another solely by the individual's ability to perceive them with his or her sensory system. In short, the differentiation between that which is form and that which is energy within any given object, plant, animal or human lies with the observer.*

✴ **Basic Sensory System Perception:** *We define basic sensory system perception as being that which the vast majority of individuals on Earth experience. The acts of* *seeing, hearing, touching, tasting and smelling fall within what we acknowledge as a basic, fundamental range of sensory development that is predominant on the Earth level. What is referred to as an "expansion experience" is, in fact, an act or experience that is perceived by an individual because of an expansion of the range in which his sensory system operates. Expansion experiences are not perceived outside or beyond an individual's electrical system, central nervous system and sensory system. These three systems are interrelated, and an accurate perception of an expansion experience requires that the three systems operate in concert. Therefore, it is quite possible for something to occur in an individual's life that registers in the person's electrical system and central nervous system but then short-circuits, is altered or is blocked simply because the person's present sensory system does not have the ability to process, due to its present range of operation, what has registered in the other two systems. People say that "these kinds of strange things never happen to me." This is inaccurate. "Strange" things, experiences and moments beyond the present state of their sensory systems, are continuously happening around them and to them. They are simply not at the point where their sensory systems are capable of clear, useful processing. They waste time by directing their will and focus to "make things happen." That is useless since things are happening all the time around them. Instead they should relax and continue through an organic developmental process that is already in effect and which will gradually allow them to accurately perceive what is happening around them. In some cases, where events or experiences are vaguely perceived*

119

or processed in outrageous, useless ways, their sensory system is expanding but still not operating within the range where events can be usefully processed.

❊ **REALITY:** *From our perspective, reality refers to all levels and dimensions of life experience within form and beyond form. Reality does not depend on an individual's perception of it in order to exist. We call an individual's perception of reality his "perceived reality." Any life system that was created in form (which occurred at the moment of the Big Bang) has inherent in it all dimensions and levels that exist both within form and beyond. How we relate to an individual or object depends on our present ability to enfold and envelop an individual's many levels. The scope within which one exists, the reality of one's existence, is truly beyond form, beyond description. If one understands that the evolutionary force which moves all life systems forward is endless—beyond time—then one must also consider that it is the continuous discovery of these vast levels inherent in all life systems that creates that evolutionary momentum. Since that dynamic is beyond time as expressed on any form level or dimension, it is endless.*

❊ **PERCEIVED REALITY:** *This is the combination of elements that make up an individual's full system of reality and are perceived, embraced and enfolded by him or by another individual at any given time. From this, an individual "knows" himself or another individual only from the perspective of the specific combination of elements he or she is able to perceive, embrace and enfold. Any one element can be considered a window to the larger whole. When in form, these*

120

elements take on the dynamics of order, organization and life vitality and are demonstrated through these specific form frameworks. The extent to which perceived reality corresponds to the larger, all-encompassing reality depends on the ability of an individual to accurately demonstrate these elements within form frameworks and the ability of that or another individual to accurately perceive what is being demonstrated.

✳ **BALANCE:** *Balance is relative and measured, shall we say, by an individual's ability to faithfully demonstrate the various elements comprising his larger reality through the specific frameworks of form in which one has chosen to develop. When what one is demonstrating is faithful in intent and clarity with these elements and the larger reality, one experiences balance. And those interacting with this individual will experience his balance. One experiences imbalance when there is distortion between what one demonstrates through the form framework and the intent and clarity of the elements comprising the larger reality as well as the larger reality itself.*

If you truly look at what we are saying here, you will see that balance as a phenomenon is not an elusive state that only an exulted few can achieve. Balance is, in fact, inherent in all reality, in all life systems. Balance is defined by the many elements within any individual's reality. And it is the dominant state of being within any reality and any form system. It is also the state of being that links individual life systems to one another and to the larger whole. When one says that he is a child of the universe, what one is acknowledging is the relationship and link of his higher state of balance to the universe's state of balance. Whether one feels linked to or distant from this relationship, depends on the closeness or distance he creates within himself with respect to his larger personal state of balance—that dynamic which is part of his overall reality.

❋ **LIFE VITALITY:** *We have used this term frequently in these definitions and feel it would be useful to clarify what we mean. To understand life vitality, it is best to see it in relationship to order and organization. Order and organization are the physical structures that create the framework for form. In short, they define the walls. But we have included the dynamic of life vitality when we refer to form because one element of form is action, and it is life vitality that initiates and creates action. Nothing in form is stagnant. It is life vitality that gives to form its action. If the framework that is created from order and organization is incomplete, ineffective, deteriorating or being dismantled in an untimely manner, the dynamic of life vitality decreases within the overall form reality. This causes life movement to decrease accordingly, and is a movement towards a state of stagnation. It is the dynamic of vitality that gives life—movement—to any individual or object. Organization and order alone cannot do that. However, vitality without organization and order has no sense of purpose to its motion. It cannot function without organization and order. The three must be present and in balance with one another for there to be quality form expression. Nature, on the devic level, creates organization, order and life vitality in perfect balance. Nature, on the nature spirit level, maintains that balanced relationship as individual life units move through their evolutionary paces.*

We would like to illustrate what we are saying by focusing your attention on the soil-balancing process that improves and enhances the level of soil vitality. This process does not work directly with the soil's vitality level. Instead, it works with those elements of the soil that comprise its order and organization. The process shores up the physical structure of its order and organization. As a direct result, the soil begins to shift its form back to the original balance among organization, order and life vitality. As a consequence of this shift, the soil vitality level (the soil's life vitality) increases to its new state of balance. Those changes involve a comparable shift in the interaction and movement among all the different elements that comprise soil. This is why when someone observes change in a field that has had its soil balanced through the soil-balancing process, he sees greater efficiency between how the soil and plants interact. The action and movement in the soil have raised the soil's order and organizational structures back to the state (or nearer to the state) of the original devic balance of order, organization and life vitality.

✳ GROUNDING: *Quite simply, the word "grounded" is used to acknowledge full body/soul fusion or full matter/soul fusion. The word "grounding" refers to what must be accomplished or activated in order to both assure and stabilize body or matter/soul fusion. To be grounded refers to the state of being a fused body (matter)/soul unit. To achieve this unit fusion and to function fully as a fused unit is the primary goal one accepts when choosing to experience life within form. Functioning as a grounded body (matter)/soul unit is a goal* on all levels and dimensions of form, whether the form can or cannot be perceived by the five senses.

Nature plays two key roles in grounding. First, it is through and with nature that the grounding occurs. Nature, which organizes, orders and adds life vitality to create form, is what creates and maintains grounding. Secondly, the levels of nature know what is required to fuse the soul dynamic within form. Nature itself provides the best examples of body (matter)/soul fusion. Humans have recognized the form or matter existence of nature on the planet, but have only recently begun to understand that within all form there are fully functioning soul dynamics. On the other hand, humans acknowledge or concentrate on their personal soul dynamics but have little understanding as to how they, in order to be functional within form, must allow the soul to fuse with and operate through their form body. Humans do not see the examples and learn the lessons of the master teachers of body (matter)/soul fusion that surround them in all the kingdoms of nature. Humans also deny the fusion within themselves. The relative extent of this denial interferes proportionately with the quality and stabilization of the fusion.

✳ **INTENT:** *Intent refers to the conscious dynamic within all life that links life vitality with soul purpose and direction. When an individual uses free will to manipulate what he or she willfully desires instead of what is within the scope of higher soul purpose, then intent is combined with the manipulative power of free will and this combination is linked with life vitality. If you will recall, it is life vitality that adds action to order and organization. It both initiates and creates* *action. To maintain harmonious movement with soul purpose and direction, life vitality must be linked with the soul dynamic. This linkage occurs on two levels. One is unconscious, allowing for a natural patterning and rhythm of action through form that is consistent with soul purpose. As the body/soul fusion moves through its own evolutionary process as a functioning unit, it takes on a greater level of consciousness and an expanded level of awareness and knowing. As a result, the unconscious link between soul dynamic and life vitality takes on a new level of operation, thus shifting it into a state of consciousness. The shift is a gradual, step-by-step evolutionary process in itself. Intent is conscious awareness of soul purpose, what is required within the scope of form to achieve soul purpose, and how the two function as a unit. Consequently, when one wishes to express soul purpose, one need only consciously fuse this purpose with appropriate form and action. This act is what is referred to when one speaks of intent.*

Intent as a dynamic is an evolutionary process in itself and, as we have said, does not suddenly envelop one's entire life fully and completely. Intent is only gradually incorporated into one's everyday life. Therefore, one does not suddenly and immediately function within the full scope of the intent dynamic in those areas of life where intent is present. Intent as a dynamic is as broad a learning arena as life itself. And in the beginning, intent can often be confused with or intermingled with free will. However, as it is developed, it becomes the cutting edge of the body/soul unit and how it operates. Intent is the key to unlimited life within the scope of form.

✻ **INTUITION:** *Intuition, as it is popularly defined, relates to a sixth sense of operation. This is false. This is not a sixth sense. When individuals experience a phenomenon that they consider to be beyond their five senses, they tend to attribute this experience to another category, the sixth sense, and call it intuition. The fact is that these expanded experiences are processed through their five senses in an expanded manner.*

Intuition, in fact, is related to and linked with intent. It is the bridge between an individual's conscious body/soul fusion—that state which he knows and understands about the body/soul fusion and how it functions—and the individual's unconscious body/soul fusion. The intuition bridges the unconscious and the conscious. This enables what is known on the level of the unconscious body/soul fusion to be incorporated with and become a part of the conscious body/soul fusion. Intuition is the communication bridge between the two which makes it possible for the conscious body/soul unit to benefit from those aspects of the unconscious body/soul unit. This benefit results when the conscious unit opens to and moves through the lessons surrounding intent. Where intent is functioning fully, these two levels, the unconscious and the conscious, are no longer separate but have become one—the expanded conscious level. Consequently, there is then no need for the bridge known as intuition.

However, lest you think otherwise, intent is not considered greater than intuition; rather, they are two excellent tools utilized equally by the highest developed souls functioning within form. We say this to caution those who read this not to think intent is "greater" than intuition and to be aimed for at the

126

exclusion of intuition. Evolution as seen from the highest perspective is endless. Therefore, discovery of all there is to know about both intuition and intent is endless. For all practical purposes, an individual can safely consider that there will never be a time in which the development of intent will be such that the need for and development of intuition will be unnecessary. As we have said, the highest souls who function to the fullest within the scope of form do so with an equal development and expansion of both intent and intuition.

These definitions were translated in July, 1990 by Machaelle Small Wright. They were translated from the nature intelligences plus Lorpuris, Hyperithon, Genesis and Universal Light.

NEW ITEMS OF INTEREST FOR MAP PEOPLE

Perelandra Paper #6: *Emergency MAP Procedure*. Step-by-step instructions on how to use MAP and work with your team during emergencies. $2

Perelandra Paper #7: *Professional MAP Teams*. For health care practitioners. How to work with a MAP team with expertise in your professional field. $2

Perelandra Paper #8: *Nature Healing Conings for Animals*. MAP is not to be used for animal healing. This paper explains how to set up a healing coning for sick and injured animals. $2

Perelandra Rose Essences II

Developed in 1992, this set of eight essences addresses the functions within the body that are activated and/or impacted during a *deep expansion experience*—such as the kind of experience one might have as a result of MAP! The essences are made from roses growing in the Perelandra garden.

Rose Essences II Set: 1/2-oz. bottles only $35

Expanded Set: Rose & Garden plus Rose Essences II.
1/2-oz. bottles $120
Dram bottles $85

Expanded Set with Book: Rose, Garden, Rose II Essences plus the book *Flower Esences*.
1/2-oz. bottles with book $128
Dram bottles with book $93

MAP ORDER FORM

___ *Behaving As If the God In All Life Mattered* $9.95

___ *Perelandra Garden Workbook* (second edition) $19.95

___ *Perelandra Garden Workbook II* $14.95

___ *Flower Essences* $10.95

___ *MAP* $9.95

___ Free catalog of all Perelandra products

Perelandra Flower Essences

___ Perelandra Rose & Garden Essences (Basic 1/2-oz. set) $90

___ Perelandra Rose & Garden Essences (Basic dram set) $65

___ Rose & Garden Essences with book *Flower Essences* (1/2 oz.) $98

___ Rose & Garden Essences with book *Flower Essences* (dram) $73

___ Perelandra Rose Essences II Set—New: 1/2-oz bottles only. $35

___ Perelandra Rose Essences Set: 1/2-oz. bottles only. $35

___ Individual Rose Essences (set 1): 1/2 oz. (check choices) $5.50

___ Gruss an Aachen	___ Ambassador
___ Peace	___ Nymphenburg
___ Eclipse	___ White Lightnin'
___ Orange Ruffles	___ Royal Highness

___ Perelandra Garden Essences Set: 1/2-oz. bottles only. $70

___ Garden Essences Set of Nine: 1/2-oz. only. (check choices) $37

___ Individual Garden Essences: 1/2-oz. (check choices) $5.50

___ Broccoli	___ Cucumber	___ Summer Squash
___ Cauliflower	___ Dill	___ Sw. Bell Pepper
___ Celery	___ Nasturtium	___ Tomato
___ Chives	___ Okra	___ Yellow Yarrow
___ Comfrey	___ Salvia	___ Zinnia
___ Corn	___ Snap Pea	___ Zucchini

___ NOTE: Please preserve my essences in vinegar instead of brandy.

Send mail order to:
Perelandra
P.O. Box 3603
Warrenton, VA 22186

Send to (please print):

Name _____

Street _____

UPS Address _____

City _____

State & Zip _____

Postage & Handling

under $6 . . 2.00

$6.01 to 10.00 . . 3.00

$10.01 to 14.00 . . 4.00

$14.01 to 25.00 . . 4.60

$25.01 to 50.00 . . 5.40

$50.01 to 75.00 . . 6.40

$75.01 to 100.00 . . 7.20

$100.01 to 150.00 . . 8.00

$150.01 and over . . 8% of order

Canadian Shipment: Please send 1-1/2 times above postage.

Subtotal: _____			
Postage & Handling: _____			
VA residents: + 4-1/2% sales tax _____			
Total: _____			

Method of Payment: ☐ Check/Money Order ☐ Visa ☐ MasterCard

Card Number: _____

Expiration Date: _____

Signature: _____

Phone: Days _____ Evenings _____

Credit card orders must be accompanied by signature.

For 24-hr. phone answering machine orders: 703/937-2153
For 24-hr. fax: 703/937-3360

Note: Prices and shipping charges subject to change without notice.